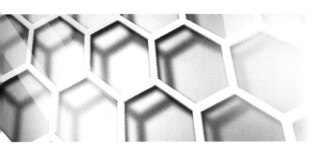

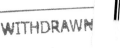
A Competency-Based Framework for Health Education Specialists – 2010

The National Commission for Health Education
Credentialing, Inc.
Society for Public Health Education
American Association for Health Education

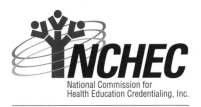

NCHEC
National Commission for
Health Education Credentialing, Inc.
Credentialing Excellence in Health Education

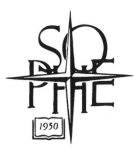

SOPHE
1950

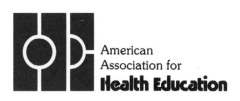

American
Association for
Health Education

A Competency-Based Framework for Health Education Specialists – 2010

For reprint permission or ordering information contact
The National Commission for Health Education Credentialing, Inc.
1541 Alta Drive, Suite 303 Whitehall, PA 18052-5642
www.nchec.org   888-624-3248

Acknowledgements

Health Educator Job Analysis Project Contributors

Optimal health is essential to quality of life. Health education specialists can significantly impact health and wellbeing when the Competencies they need to support individual and population health are clearly delineated and effectively developed. The National Health Educator Job Analysis 2010 (HEJA 2010) is the latest in the evolution of health education Competencies, which underlie the profession's commitment to excellence in health education teaching, research and practice.

The National Commission for Health Education Credentialing Inc. (NCHEC), the Society for Public Health Education (SOPHE), and the American Association for Health Education (AAHE), are joint copyright holders of this document, the HEJA 2010 Technical Report, and the project data. As such, the leaders of these three organizations wish to express their deep appreciation to several key individuals. First, our thanks goes to Eva Doyle, PhD, MSEd, CHES, who chaired the HEJA 2010 Task Force and devoted thousands of hours to guiding its conceptualization, implementation, data analysis and interpretation. Without Eva's insights, leadership and attention to detail, a project of this magnitude would not have been completed in such a timely and efficient fashion. We also wish to express our sincere thanks to Carla M. Caro, MA, and Patricia M. Muenzen, MA, of the Professional Examination Service (PES) of New York, a nonprofit credentialing and competency assurance organization contracted to assist with the project. Their expertise, professionalism, and dedication to this initiative are deeply appreciated.

The copyright holders also acknowledge the contribution of a large number of volunteers who invested time and effort in this endeavor. These volunteers, whose names are listed in Appendix C, include professionals who served in various roles related to study procedures and who contributed in some way to the development of this publication.

Deep appreciation is also extended to the dedicated health education specialists who invested time and effort into completing the HEJA 2010 survey, as well as hundreds of professional volunteers who contributed in various ways to the work described in this book.

Contributors to *A Competency-Based Framework for Health Education Specialists – 2010*

Editor

Eva Doyle, PhD, MSEd, CHES

Contributing Authors

Chris Arthur, PhD, CHES
Donna Beal, MPH, CHES
Cam Escoffery, PhD, MPH, CHES
Patricia A. Frye, DrPH, MPA, CHES

Melissa Grim, PhD, CHES
Leonard Jack, Jr., PhD, MSc, CHES
Dennis Kamholtz, PhD, CHES
Maurice "Bud" Martin, PhD, CHES
Beverly Saxton Mahoney, RN, MS, PhD, CHES
James McKenzie, MPH, PhD, CHES
Angela Mickalide, PhD, CHES
Jacquie Rainey, PhD, CHES
Rebecca Reeve, PhD, CHES
Christopher N. Thomas, MS, CHES
Tung-Sung "Sam" Tseng, DrPH, MS, CHES
Kelly Wilson, PhD, CHES
Katherine Wilson, PhD, CHES

Reviewers

M. Elaine Auld, MPH, CHES
Carla M. Caro, MA
Linda Lysoby, MS, CHES, CAE
Beverly Saxton Mahoney, RN, MS, PhD, CHES
Becky J. Smith, PhD, CHES, CAE
Patricia M. Muenzen, MA
Laura Rasar King, MPH, CHES
Alyson Taub, PhD, CHES

Copy Editors

Melissa Rehrig, MPH, CHES
Jeff Housman, PhD, CHES
Emily Glazer, MS, CHES

The format and some content of this book was based on *A Competency-Based Framework for Health Educators 2006.*
Writers of that publication included:

Stephen Stewart, PhD, CHES
Donna Videto, PhD, CHES
Tom Butler, PhD, CHES
Susan Radius, PhD, CHES

Table of Contents

Table of Contents

Introduction

The purpose of this publication is to communicate the Responsibilities, Competencies and Sub-competencies that are essential to health education practice. This document contains descriptions of the processes, outcomes, and related materials of the most recent update project known as the National Health Educator Job Analysis 2010 (HEJA 2010). It is designed for use by the health education profession as a framework for professional preparation, credentialing, and professional development.

Section I contains a brief overview of historical perspectives related to the growth and evolution of the health education profession. In Section II, the processes and outcomes of HEJA 2010 are described. The resulting HEJA 2010 model containing the updated Areas of Responsibility, Competencies, and Sub-competencies for a health education specialist is presented in Section III. Section IV contains recommended uses of the HEJA 2010 Model for various stakeholders and a set of six specific recommendations for the profession. Section V contains a comparison of the HEJA 2010 Model with the former model produced in the Competencies Update Project (CUP). Section VI contains a set of knowledge items validated in the HEJA 2010 analysis as useful in the practice of health education. Additional materials that can be used to master professional terminology and adapt professional preparation and development efforts to the HEJA 2010 Model are included in the appendices. ◆

Section I:
Historical Perspectives

Section I: Historical Perspectives

The National Health Educator Job Analysis 2010 (HEJA 2010) emerged as part of a historically-strong vision among health educators to continually embrace contemporary practice and lead others into the future. This pioneer spirit is evident within the historical perspectives described below. This section contains an overview of the first role delineation project and its impact on professional preparation and certification; the development of graduate-level Competencies; the follow-up development of the Competencies Update Project (CUP) Model (Airhihenbuwa et al., 2005) and its implications for individual certification; and emerging trends in job analysis that led to the implementation of the HEJA 2010.

Role Delineation

The history of health education in the United States dates back to the late 19th century with the establishment of the first academic programs preparing school health educators (Allegrante et al., 2004). Interest in quality assurance and the development of standards for professional preparation of health education specialists emerged in the 1940s. Over the next several decades, professional associations produced guidelines for preparing health education specialists and accreditation efforts were introduced. Yet, it was not until the 1970s that health education began evolving as a true profession (Livingood & Auld, 2001). In addition to defining a body of literature, efforts were initiated to promulgate a health education code of ethics, agreed upon use of terminology, a skill-based set of competencies, rigorous systems for quality assurance, and a health education credentialing system.

Long-standing questions about what health educators do in practice eventually led to the first Role Delineation Project in the 1970s. In February 1978, the First Bethesda Conference assembled health educators from all practice settings to begin the process of defining and verifying the role of health educators. The stated purposes of the conference were to analyze the commonalities and differences that existed in the preparation of health educators for different practice settings and to determine the potential for developing acceptable guidelines for professional preparation that would include all practice settings (NCHEC, 1985). The conference's recommendation to establish the National Task Force on the Preparation and Practice of Health Educators was realized in March 1978. This task force, in collaboration with the National Center for Health Education, undertook the landmark Role Delineation Project (United States Department of Health, Education, and Welfare, 1978).

After considerable public discussion and background research, the role of the entry-level health educator was defined during the years 1978 to 1981. Responsibilities, functions, skills, and knowledge expected of the entry-level health educator were delineated. The national survey of practicing health educators verified and refined the definition. Leaders of that project discovered that there was a "generic role" of all health educators; that is, there are commonalities in the roles and functions of entry-level health educators regardless of whether they are employed in schools, communities, worksites, or other settings. This finding formed the basis for credentialing health educators and academic programs in health education.

Professional Preparation and Certification

Using the defined role, the National Task Force on the Preparation and Practice of Health Educators developed a curriculum framework from 1981 to 1985. This framework was based on contributions from academics and practitioners involved in two national conferences, several regional workshops, and many meetings of professional associations. The resulting document, *A Framework for the Development of Competency-Based Curricula for Entry-Level Health Educators* (NCHEC, 1985), provided professional preparation programs a frame of reference for developing their health education curricula. A Competency was defined as "an ability to apply a certain specified skill in dealing with some defined amount of meaningful subject matter" (NCHEC, 1985, p. 2). As such, Competencies were viewed as a reflection of both content and process.

The Second Bethesda Conference in 1986 provided consensus that a certification process was appropriate to ensure that individuals delivering health education services possessed a minimal level of competency. Preliminary steps for developing a national certification system for health educators were initiated, culminating with the establishment of the National Commission for Health Education Credentialing (NCHEC) in 1988. Following a charter certification phase in 1989, during which individuals who met eligibility requirements could become certified through a review of documentation submitted (e.g., letters of support, academic records), the first national competency-based certification examination was offered by NCHEC in 1990. Thus, the Competencies identified through this role delineation process formed the basis for a framework for professional preparation and a national examination, leading to credentialing the eligible individual as a Certified Health Education Specialist (CHES) (NCHEC, 1996).

Graduate-Level Competencies

Efforts to determine graduate-level Competencies were initiated in 1992 by the American Association for Health Education (AAHE) and the Society for Public Health Education (SOPHE), which commissioned the Joint Committee for the Development of Graduate-Level Preparation Standards. The committee sought the input of academics involved in graduate-level professional preparation through a national survey and at various annual meetings, as well as through its own continuing deliberations, to ascertain the advanced-level Competencies practiced by health educators with advanced training and experience. It was projected that such Competencies would build on the entry-level skills within the Seven Areas of Responsibility that had been identified, as well as establish new Areas of Responsibility at the advanced-levels.

Following the publication of a final report and its acceptance by the boards of AAHE, NCHEC, and SOPHE, the Graduate Competencies Implementation Committee was formed (SOPHE & AAHE, 1997). This committee addressed the manner in which the new advanced-level Competencies would be disseminated to, and implemented by, the profession. The resulting document, *A Competency-Based Framework for Graduate-Level Health Education Specialists*, was jointly published in 1999 by AAHE, NCHEC, and SOPHE (AAHE, NCHEC, & SOPHE, 1999). This publication contained a complete history of the development of the proposed advanced-level Competencies.

The CUP Model

During the mid- to-late 1990s, professional organizations and individual health educators expressed a desire to re-verify the entry-level Competencies to ensure that they reflected current health education research findings and practice; to further integrate, refine, and validate the advanced (graduate-level) Competencies; and to add to the advanced Competencies as appropriate. To this end, NCHEC initiated the National Health Educator Competencies Update Project (CUP) in 1998, with the participation of AAHE, SOPHE, and nine other national health education–related organizations. This six-year (1998-2004), multiphase national research study was guided by the CUP National Advisory Committee, consisting of representatives of the 12 national professional groups, and a CUP Steering Committee that led the project with assistance from research experts (Gilmore, Olsen, Taub, & Connell, 2005). The project included a planning and resource-development phase (1998-1999), a survey development and pilot process (2000-2001), and a four-year data collection, analysis, and reporting phase (2001-2004).

Seven updated Areas of Responsibility, 35 Competencies, and 163 Sub-competencies emerged from the study (Gilmore, Olsen, Taub, & Connell, 2005). Three levels of practice defined by years of experience and degrees were also identified:

- ***Entry-level:*** less than five years of experience with a baccalaureate or master's degree
- ***Advanced 1-level:*** five or more years of experience with a baccalaureate or master's degree
- ***Advanced 2-level:*** five or more years of experience with a doctoral degree

Though health educators at all three levels practiced some aspects of all Seven Areas of Responsibility, small subsets of Competencies and Sub-competencies were identified as unique to the advanced-levels. The CUP research revealed three distinct levels of practice, each building on the others, from entry to advanced. For this reason, a new hierarchical model, the CUP Model, emerged from the research findings. The CUP Model had implications for professional preparation, credentialing, and professional development (Gilmore, Olsen, Taub, & Connell, 2005).

As a result of the CUP research, SOPHE, AAHE and NCHEC issued a set of four recommendations to the profession in 2005. Among the recommendations were that baccalaureate programs in health education prepare their graduates to perform all Seven Areas of Responsibility and the Competencies/Sub-competencies specified as entry-level in the CUP hierarchical model. Similarly, it was recommended that graduate programs in health education prepare their graduates to perform all Seven Areas of Responsibility and the Competencies/Sub-competencies in the CUP Model at the advanced-levels as appropriate to the degree level. Also, a recommendation was made to NCHEC to use the Seven Areas of Responsibility, Competencies, and Sub-competencies identified as entry-level as the basis for revising the entry-level certification examination (Airhihenbuwa et al., 2005).

The CUP Model and recommendations were subsequently endorsed in 2006 by all member organizations of the Coalition of National Health Education Organizations (CNHEO), a coalition of nine professional organizations of which health educators are members. At the Third National Congress for Institutions Preparing Health Education Specialists: Linking Program Assessment, Accountability and Improvement in February 2006, information about the CUP Model and findings were made available for the first time through plenary presentations, workshops, and the official release of a new edition of *A Competency-Based Framework for Health Educators* (NCHEC, SOPHE, & AAHE, 2006).

Competency-Based Accreditation

As the CUP investigation was beginning to take shape, AAHE and SOPHE convened an invitational meeting in 2000 of key health education leaders to explore various issues facing the profession in quality assurance, including a fragmented system of program approval processes and accreditation mechanisms (Allegrante et al., 2004). A critical recommendation from the meeting was that "a comprehensive, coordinated accreditation system for undergraduate and graduate health education should be put into place, which builds on the strengths of current mechanisms" (Allegrante et al., 2004, p. 672). Subsequently, a three-year (2001-2003) task force, known as the National Task Force on Accreditation in Health Education, developed principles and seven recommendations for strengthening both professional preparation and certification in health education. In 2004, AAHE and SOPHE commissioned the next phase (2004-2006) of this work known as the National Transition Task Force on Accreditation in Health Education to help implement the recommendations. In 2006, this task force convened in Dallas, TX, the Third National Congress for Institutions Preparing Health Educators, a landmark meeting sometimes referred to as Dallas II because the earlier congress of 1996 designed to discuss graduate-level Competencies was also in Dallas (the first congress was in Birmingham, AL, in 1981) (Taub, Birch, Auld, Lysoby, & Rasar King, 2009).

The Dallas II meeting, sponsored by SOPHE and AAHE, drew together over 250 university faculty and administrators from over 150 professional preparation programs (Taub, Birch, Auld, Lysoby, & Rasar King, 2009). The purpose of Dallas II was to provide an update of the effort to establish a unified system of accreditation for the health education profession, review and discuss future accreditation developments, disseminate and discuss the implications of the new CUP Model, and identify issues and strategies for the transition to a unified accreditation system.

According to Taub, Birch, Auld, Lysoby, and Rasar King (2009), accreditation discussions focused on potential avenues for transitioning to a more unified system. AAHE had partnered since 1988 with the National Council for Accreditation of Teacher Education (NCATE), the officially-recognized accrediting body for professional preparation programs in school health education. The Council on Education for Public Health (CEPH) had been accrediting master-level public health schools and programs since 1978 (a process originally established and maintained by the American Public Health Association in the early 1970s). CEPH had begun to accredit baccalaureate public or community health education programs linked to graduate public health programs and schools, but had not been accrediting free-standing baccalaureate public/community health education programs (CEPH, 2005). SOPHE established in 1980, and was joined by AAHE in 1984, an approval process for baccalaureate public or community health education programs through the SOPHE/AAHE Baccalaureate Approval Committee (SABPAC). SABPAC approval was based on the Competencies of a health educator and included a peer review process for self-study using assessment criteria; however, the lack of an official accreditation status for the SABPAC has been a challenge.

The Dallas II discussion revolved around the possibility of CEPH becoming the accrediting body for all professional preparation programs in community health education, regardless of their affiliation status with graduate-level public health schools and programs (Taub, Birch, Auld, Lysoby, & Rasar King, 2009). Challenges were discussed as they related to differences in terminology regarding a "unified" versus a "coordinated" multiple-body accrediting system, potential philosophical differences between public and community health, and capacity challenges for small professional preparation programs that would need to be accredited.

Further exploration into accreditation possibilities was deemed important. Following the Dallas II meeting, SOPHE and AAHE established the National Implementation Task Force for Accreditation in Health Education in 2007. Meanwhile, the CUP Model replaced the original Responsibilities and Competencies from the Role Delineation Project in the SABPAC approval requirements (SOPHE & AAHE, 2007). The CUP Model and any further development of professional Competencies would need to be an essential part of future accreditation discussions with CEPH leaders and other stakeholders (Taub, Birch, Auld, Lysoby, & Rasar King, 2009). Unifying the profession on accreditation for professional preparation would also require a unified acceptance and application of established Competencies for individual certification and health education practice.

Implications for Individual Certification

The dissemination and endorsement of the new CUP Model initiated changes in the structure of the CHES exam for entry-level health educators and discussions about the possible need for an advanced-level certification. NCHEC leaders adapted the examination blueprint framework for the certification exam questions, released a new study guide, and launched the first examination based on the CUP Model outcomes in the fall of 2007 (NCHEC, 2007). Performance rates on the new exam were comparable to previous performance rates (Dennis & Mahoney, 2008). This validated beliefs that the primary components of the CUP Model were not only reflective of contemporary practice, but also the professional preparation programs that are often shaped by contemporary practice.

CUP findings regarding advanced-levels of practice held significant implications for NCHEC and the profession. The development and maintenance of an advanced-level certification would be costly and complex for a number of reasons. The fact that two advanced-levels were identified in the CUP heightened the need to be deliberate and thorough in designing an appropriate action plan. Part of the challenge in developing advanced-level certification rested in the smaller number of advanced-level Competencies and Sub-competencies resulting from the CUP.

Despite these limitations, the exciting prospect and potential benefits of instituting an advanced-level credential was compelling. The CUP findings indicated the need to take initial steps in that direction. The results of an NCHEC-sponsored survey of stakeholders, and further discussions with multiple national leadership groups, were also supportive of moving ahead. Additionally, creating distinct levels of certification was in line with one of the recommendations of the National Task Force on Accreditation in Health Education (Allegrante et al., 2004). These factors and feasibility deliberations among various NCHEC working groups led NCHEC leaders to announce in the fall of 2008 its plans to develop an advanced-level of certification. Following a period of public comment about such issues as eligibility criteria and certification mechanisms, the NCHEC Board of Commissioners issued in May of 2009 a policy statement regarding a new advanced-level credential (NCHEC, 2009). The new credential would be called the Master Certified Health Education Specialist (MCHES). MCHES eligibility would be aligned with CUP findings regarding delineation of five years of experience and based on a combination of entry- and advanced-level Competencies and Sub-competencies.

Emerging Trends in Job Analyses

In the midst of these developments toward advanced-level certification, NCHEC leaders also received news of an organizational achievement that would significantly impact future approaches to competencies research updates. In June of 2008, the CHES certification was granted accreditation by the National Commission for Certifying Agencies (NCCA), the accreditation body of the Institute for Credentialing Excellence that accredits professional certification organizations (ICE, 2009). Obtaining a *gold standard* endorsement by the leading body in testing accreditation made a profound statement within the national credentialing industry about the quality of the CHES exam and its reflection of a clearly-defined profession (NCHEC, 2008).

Among the NCCA *Standards for the Accreditation of Certification Programs* is the requirement that a professional role delineation or job analysis be conducted and periodically validated (ICE, 2009). A number of accrediting bodies require leaders of professional preparation programs to submit data-based documents for review every five years (CEPH, 2005; SOPHE & AAHE, 2007). The challenge of this five-year cycle lies in developing a system that allows program leaders to collect and analyze data, interpret findings in light of goals and existing frameworks, and make adjustments based on identified trends; however, the potential benefits can outweigh these challenges for a profession in the midst of rapid development.

As can be noted in Figure 1.1, the health education profession has been in a stage of relatively constant growth and change since the 1970s. More recent changes and emerging workforce issues have included the already-mentioned movement toward a more unified accreditation system along with discussions about competency frameworks for health promotion in international settings, the emergence of a general (non-health education specific) certification in public health, and a projected downshift in school-based jobs balanced by high growth in community and public health settings (Battel-Kirk, Barry, Taub, & Lysoby, 2009; Bureau of Labor Statistics, 2007; Cottrell et al., 2009; Howze, Auld, Woodhouse, Gershick, & Livingood, 2009).

The six-year CUP study had produced an invaluable foundation for the profession in that it identified and validated the essential elements of professional practice in health education including guidelines for the development of advanced-levels. Based on recommendations from the NCCA and certification industry standards for staying abreast of contemporary trends in the profession, the next step entailed the need to again verify the Responsibilities, Competencies, and Sub-competencies used in practice. The methods and timeframe of this job analysis would need to be effectively streamlined to meet the five-year cycle. NCHEC consulted with representatives of NCCA and the Professional Examination Service (PES), a national testing corporation that works with NCHEC to oversee the CHES examination process. These experts advised leaders of NCHEC, SOPHE, and AAHE about best-practice standards and industry norms related to job analyses. PES representatives created a research design for the needed job analysis that was based on industry-accepted procedures. This analysis, the HEJA 2010, was launched in 2008 and completed in 2009. Descriptions of HEJA 2010 procedures and methods, outcomes, and recommendations are included in this publication. The results of the HEJA 2010 have implications for certification, accreditation, professional preparation and professional development.

Figure 1.1
Historical Time Line of
Selected Milestones

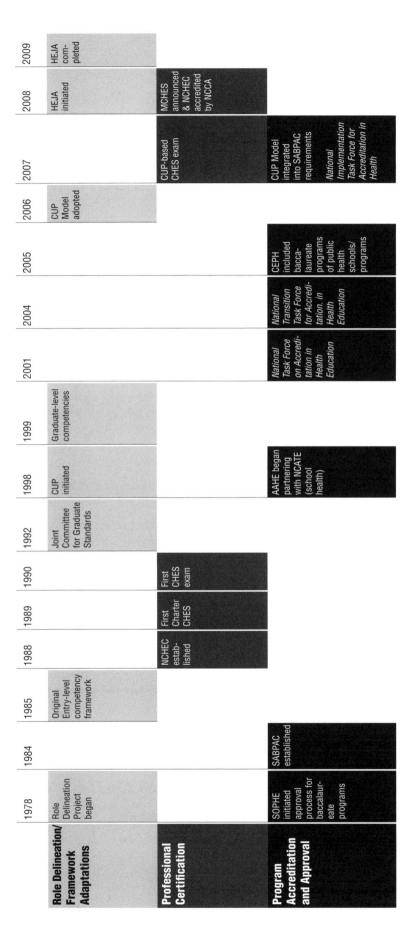

	1978	1984	1985	1988	1989	1990	1992	1998	1999	2001	2004	2005	2006	2007	2008	2009
Role Delineation/ Framework Adaptations	Role Delineation Project began		Original Entry-level competency framework				Joint Committee for Graduate Standards	CUP initiated	Graduate-level competencies				CUP Model adopted		HEJA initiated	HEJA completed
Professional Certification				NCHEC established	First Charter CHES	First CHES exam								CUP-based CHES exam	MCHES announced & NCHEC accredited by NCCA	
Program Accreditation and Approval	SOPHE initiated approval process for baccalaureate programs	SABPAC established						AAHE began partnering with NCATE (school health)		*National Task Force on Accreditation in Health Education*	*National Transition Task Force for Accreditation in Health Education*	CEPH included baccalaureate programs of public health schools/ programs		CUP Model integrated into SABPAC requirements *National Implementation Task Force for Accreditation in Health*		

Section II:
HEJA 2010 Process
and Outcomes

Section II: HEJA 2010 Process and Outcomes

The National Health Educator Job Analysis 2010 (HEJA 2010) was implemented to validate the contemporary practice of entry- and advanced-level health education specialists. Findings would be used to develop the examinations for a Certified Health Education Specialist (CHES) and a Master Certified Health Education Specialist (MCHES), report validated changes in health education practice since the CUP study, and inform professional preparation and continuing education initiatives. The study was initiated in 2008 to meet accreditation standards of the National Commission for Certifying Agencies (NCCA), which requires regular, periodic re-verification of the competencies upon which the credential is based.

Job analysis experts from Professional Examination Services (PES) designed and conducted the study. These PES experts based their approach on credentialing industry standards and best-practices guidelines established by the American Educational Research Association (AERA), American Psychological Association (APA), and National Council on Measurement in Education (NCME), as well as other recognized sources for practice analysis updates (Hambleton & Rogers, 1986; NCCA, 2005; Raymond, 2002).

HEJA 2010 Participants

The HEJA 2010 study, under the direction of PES, was guided by two groups of health education professionals: the 2010 Health Education Job Analysis Steering Committee (HEJA 2010-SC) and the 2010 Health Education Job Analysis Task Force (HEJA 2010-TF). The HEJA 2010-SC consisted of the chief staff officers from each sponsoring organization, the 2008 coordinator of the NCHEC Division Board for Certification of Health Education Specialists, and the appointed HEJA 2010-TF chair. The 11 HEJA 2010-TF members were selected from a pool of more than 200 volunteer nominees generated through a call to the profession. An additional 48 volunteers selected from this pool served in the instrument development phase of the study as subject-matter experts (n=9), independent reviewers (n=18), and survey pilot participants (n=21). These 59 volunteers were selected to ensure representation of the diversity of health education work settings, educational backgrounds, and experience levels; and to maintain demographic and geographic diversity.

In the survey implementation phase of the study, a primary goal in the sampling process was to achieve representation among survey participants from all work settings, education levels, years of experience, and CHES status. Because no single source exists through which all practicing health education specialists can be accessed, multiple approaches were used to develop the sample of health education specialists invited to complete the survey. Member organizations of the Coalition of National Health Education Organizations (CNHEO) helped publicize the study to their members via electronic communication channels and conferences. These communications included a link to an online site where volunteers could sign up to participate and provide their e-mail address to which a survey link could be sent.

Nine hundred eighteen volunteers responded to invitations disseminated through CNHEO members. In addition, a stratified random sampling technique was used to draw a sample of 4,208 Certified Health Education Specialists (CHES) from the NCHEC database that represented all work settings and varying years of experience. An invitation to complete the online survey was e-mailed to this total de-duped sample of 5,126 health education specialists. Of the 5,126 e-mail addresses to which invitations were sent, 269 were invalid. Another 108 individuals on this list were removed from the database based on an initial screening to include only practicing health education specialists as participants. Of the resulting 4,749 practicing health education specialists sampled, 1,022 completed the survey for a response rate of 21.5%. Responding health education specialists were distributed across 49 states and the District of Columbia and a wide array of work settings (e.g., community, school, college/university, health care, business/industry).

HEJA 2010 Procedures

The 18-month HEJA 2010 study (June 2008 to November 2009) entailed the process of selecting volunteers previously described, followed by two general phases of instrument development and implementation. In the instrument development phase, a combination of structured interviews, focus groups, and modified Delphi techniques was used to systematically update the model of health education practice and to create and refine a survey instrument. The survey was disseminated to the sample described above for validation of the updated model by practicing health education specialists. Data were collected and the results were analyzed and interpreted. The entire 18-month study process consisted of the following steps (see Figure 2.1):

1. *Volunteer selection:* Selection of the HEJA 2010-TF and other volunteer health education specialists to contribute to instrument development (June–July 2008)
2. *Telephone interviews:* Preliminary telephone interviews with 9 subject matter experts (August 2008)
3. *Task force meeting #1:* Preliminary work by the HEJA 2010-TF to update the description of health education practice through a face-to-face meeting and follow-up activities (September–October 2008)
4. *Terminology review:* Follow-up work of a terminology committee (3 HEJA 2010-TF members) to review the draft survey for consistency of terms (November 2008)
5. *Task force review:* A Web-based HEJA 2010-TF review of and comment on the draft survey (December 2008)
6. *Content reconciliation:* Follow-up work of a content reconciliation committee (2 HEJA 2010-TF members and 1 steering committee member) to reconcile feedback from individual HEJA 2010-TF members (December 2008)
7. *Independent review:* An independent review process with 18 independent reviewers representing diverse work settings (December 2008–January 2009)
8. *Task force meeting #2:* A face-to-face meeting of the HEJA 2010-TF to review and reconcile the independent review results, create a pre-survey iteration of the model, and develop survey rating scales (January 2009)
9. *Sampling plan development:* Development of a stratified random sampling plan for the validation survey by PES, and outreach to the profession for volunteer survey participants by CNHEO member organizations (January 2009)
10. *Institutional review board approval:* Institutional Review Board approval of the study by Baylor University (February 2009)

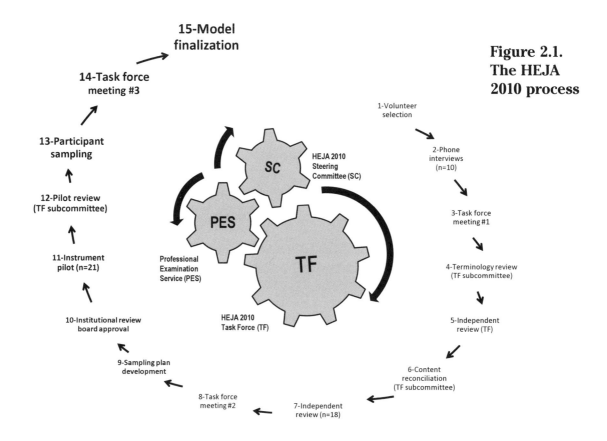

**Figure 2.1.
The HEJA
2010 process**

11. *Instrument pilot:* Pilot testing of the online survey instrument for comprehensiveness, clarity, and technical ease of use by 21 pilot testers (February 2009)

12. *Pilot review:* HEJA 2010-TF subcommittee review and reconciliation based upon pilot test findings (March 2009)

13. *Participant sampling:* E-mail invitations to participate in the survey sent to a valid sample of 4,749 health education specialists. Periodic reminders sent throughout 4-week completion window, resulting in 1,022 responses, a 21.5% response rate (April–May 2009)

14. *Task force meeting #3:* HEJA 2010-TF review of survey results in a face-to-face meeting and development of recommendations to the HEJA 2010-SC (June 2009)

15. *Model finalization:* HEJA 2010-SC review of task force recommendations and finalization of the model (July–November 2009)

Conceptual framework for instrument development

As illustrated in Figure 2.1, the HEJA 2010-TF played a critical and continuous decision-making role throughout the job analysis. The task force first developed an updated model of Areas of Responsibility, Competencies, and Sub-competencies to be used in an analysis of practice in the national survey. A modified Delphi technique (Ali, 2005; Benarie, 1988; Gilmore & Campbell, 2005; Woudenberg, 1991) was used in a series of steps (Steps 3-12 of Figure 2.1) for model development. The task force created the first iteration of the model in Step 3 and, then, systematically reviewed feedback from various working groups and gradually developed and refined the model for use as a survey instrument in Steps four through 12. Throughout this process, the task force integrated into its decision-making the input provided by other HEJA 2010 work groups, guidelines from PES regarding competency development, and recommendations and emerging professional trends evident in the following sources:

CUP: Results of the National Health Educator Competencies Update Project [CUP] (NCHEC, SOPHE, & AAHE, 2006).

Crosswalk: Recommendations were submitted to the HEJA 2010-TF from leaders of the Coalition of National Health Education Organizations (CNHEO) who recently completed the "Crosswalk Project." In this project, leaders examined similarities and differences in the health education Competencies used in the CHES exam with the public health competencies that frame the Certified in Public Health exam (Woodhouse et al., 2010).

Health Education Terminology: Guidelines for health education terminology (Joint Committee on Terminology, 2001).

The Galway Consensus Conference Statement: A consensus statement on core competencies for building global capacity in health promotion that emerged from an international conference in Galway, Ireland, in June of 2008 (Allegrante et al., 2009).

Marketing the Health Education Profession: A study commissioned by CNHEO and other leading organizations to examine employers' knowledge, attitudes and hiring practices of health educator employers (Hezel Associates, 2007; Gambescia et al., 2009).

Recommendations from the Final Report of The National Task Force on Accreditation in Health Education regarding graduate professional preparation and the need for a master-level certification for health education specialist were also important considerations (Allegrante et al., 2004; Taub, Birch, Auld, Lysoby, & Rasar King, 2009). The resulting model was adapted to an online survey format, and used in the national validation survey.

In the early stages of updating Competencies and Sub-competencies for use in the study, members of the task force sometimes found themselves discussing the types and depth of knowledge a health education specialist would need to possess to effectively perform a specific Competency or Sub-competency. This discussion arose most frequently within the context of the long-range use of study outcomes to shape professional preparation and development efforts. Though task force members agreed that a competency-based approach to professional preparation, credentialing, and on-going development is essential, the group also recognized the utility of identifying relevant knowledge bases that should be included in professional preparation and development efforts.

For this reason, the task force decided to include a knowledge-based survey in the study. The same modified Delphi technique used to develop the updated competency model was also used to develop 115 knowledge items for use in the HEJA 2010 survey. The PES experts created a 4-point rating scale for the knowledge items that was based on the Revised Bloom's Taxonomy (Anderson & Krathwohl, 2001) of remembering, understanding, applying, analyzing, evaluating, and creating knowledge. Because this was the first time in the history of job analyses conducted for the health education profession that knowledge items were included, the process used to develop and validate the knowledge items is considered a pilot study.

Survey instrument

The model of health education practice presented to survey participants via the instrument used for the validation survey included 246 Sub-competencies framed within eight Areas (evaluation and research Sub-competencies were formatted within separate Areas for purposes of this study). The 4-point rating scales used in the Competencies Update Project (CUP) (NCHEC, SOPHE, & AAHE, 2006) completed in 2005 were used in this instrument to ensure comparability of results, and participants rated each Sub-competency in terms of:

- Frequency of practice within the past 12 months: *Not at all, occasionally (less than once a month), frequently (at least once each month) very frequently (at least once each week)*
- Importance of the Sub-competency to the participant's work: *Not important, minimally important, moderately important, highly important*

The instrument also contained 115 knowledge items. A 4-point rating scale based on the Revised Bloom's Taxonomy was used by participants to rate these items in terms of cognitive levels of use in their work (*I do not use the knowledge, I recognize and/or recall the knowledge, I apply and/or integrate the knowledge, I use the knowledge to evaluate and/or create*). Demographic and professional questions were included to gather information about participant education, experience level, work setting, type of work performed, professional credentials, organizational memberships, gender, and race/ethnicity.

As previously indicated, the online survey was tested through a survey pilot. Based on pilot feedback, the online survey system was adjusted to allow participants to exit and return to the system as needed over time to complete the full survey. Upon entry into the online survey system, participants were directed to read a study overview and indicate *informed consent* (approved by an institutional review board) prior to completing the one-hour survey.

Analysis and Outcomes

PES experts compiled survey responses, performed data reduction and analysis, and guided the HEJA 2010-TF in interpretation of the results. Demographic profiles of participants (group percentages) were developed in accordance with responses related to certification status, educational degrees earned, years of experience, work setting, geographic location, ethnicity, and gender. Work settings, years of experience, and education levels were used for subgroup analyses.

Based on an in-depth review of analysis results, the task force determined that the criteria used in the CUP (NCHEC, SOPHE, & AAHE, 2006) to validate Sub-competencies and identify practice levels were a logical and useful fit for this study. Thus, a composite score [(frequency – 1) + importance] was generated for each Sub-competency to represent a combined score for frequency and importance, and items with composite scores of 3.0 or higher were included in the model. The three levels of practice (see Table 2.1) used to analyze survey responses were based on a combination of experience and education level: entry (less than five years of experience and a baccalaureate or master's degree), advanced 1 (five or more years of experience and a baccalaureate or master's degree), and advanced 2 (five or more years of experience and a doctoral degree).

Table 2.1
Practice levels for health education specialists

Level of Practice	Definition	Competencies & Sub-competencies
Entry	Less than 5 years of experience Baccalaureate or master's degree	Entry
Advanced 1	5 or more years of experience Baccalaureate or master's degree	Entry + Advanced 1
Advanced 2	5 or more years of experience Doctoral degree	Entry + Advanced 1 + Advanced 2

Knowledge items were included in a national survey for the first time in the history of job analyses in the health education profession. Knowledge-related survey items were validated for inclusion in a knowledge list if at least 50% of participants indicated use of that knowledge at some cognitive level. Demographic information about study participants and more details about instrument development and study outcomes are provided below.

Demographics

One thousand twenty-two of the 4,749 practicing health education specialists sampled completed the survey. This overall response rate of 21.5% was consistent with the range of response rates generally found in professional job analyses (Impara, 1995). Of the 1,022 participants, 72% were CHES randomly sampled from the NCHEC data base (n=739). The remaining 283 participants were CHES (n=160, 16% of total sample) and non-CHES (n=123, 12% of total sample) volunteers who responded to invitations through professional organizations. The response rates for these three subgroups were 46.4% (160 of 345) for CHES volunteers, 22.1% (123 of 557) for non-CHES volunteers, and 19.2% (739 of 3847) for CHES randomly sampled from the NCHEC database.

Forty-nine states, the District of Columbia, and Puerto Rico were represented in the respondent pool. The states with the largest number of participants were California (98, 11.0% of total), Texas (47, 5.3%), Georgia (45, 5.1%), and Pennsylvania (43, 4.8%). Of the 990 participants who indicated a race/ethnicity category, the following categories were checked: White or Caucasian (76.7%), Black or African American (11.7%), Hispanic or Latino/Latina (4.9%), Asian (3.3%), Multi-ethnic (2.4%), American Indian or Alaska Native (.7%), Other (.2%). Of the 998 participants who indicated their gender, 87.5% were female.

The participants were relatively experienced, with a mean of 13.1 years of work experience and an average of 5.9 years spent in their current position. Just over 78% had worked for 5 or more years. For the highest degree earned, 194 (19.0%) had earned a baccalaureate degree, 658 (64.4%) had earned a master's degree, and 170 (16.6%) had earned a doctoral degree. Based on the established definitions for levels of practice, 210 (21%) of participants were entry-level, 647 (65%) participants were advanced 1-level, and 139 (14%) were advanced 2-level. Half of all participants were advanced 1-level health education specialists with a master's degree.

Of the 1,022 participants, 1,011 responded to a survey item in which they indicated one of the eight work setting categories as their primary work setting (see Table 2.2). The majority of these respondents indicated they worked in government (26.2%), university-based academia (16.6%), health care (16.1%), and community (15.0%) settings. When subgrouped by practice level, 65.6% of entry-level respondents (n=209) worked in government (26.3%), community (21.1%), and health care (18.2%) settings. Among the 646 advanced-level respondents, 62.5% worked in government (29.7%), and health care (17.5%), and community (15.3%), settings. A significant shift in work setting representation was evident among the 139 advanced 2-level respondents in that 61.9% worked in an academic setting (as a university faculty member) and 13.7% worked in college or university health services (e.g., student wellness programs or health clinics).

Table 2.2

Work settings of survey participants

Work Setting	n	%

Community
    Health planning agency
    Voluntary health agency
    Non-profit health education center
    Non-profit health organization
	152	15.0%

Government
    Municipal, county or district health department
    State health department
    Federal government agency
	265	26.2%

School
    Elementary and/or secondary school
    State education department
	67	6.6%

Business
    Business or industry
    Organized labor
	67	6.6%

Health care
    Hospital
    Non-hospital health care facility
    Managed care organization or health plan
	163	16.1%

Academia College or university	168	16.6%
College Health University or college health services	75	7.4%

Other
    Professional association
    Self-employed
    Military
    Other
	54	5.3%

Total	**1,011***	**100%**

Note. Of 1,022 participants, 1,011 provided work-setting information

SECTION: II

Generic Sub-competencies

The composite score [(frequency – 1) + importance] generated for each Sub-competency represented a stronger weighting for the *importance* of a Sub-competency to the job, in relation to the frequency with which it was practiced. This weighting was based on the rationale that, even if not frequently performed, a Sub-competency could still be important; however, a Sub-competency would be dropped or excluded from the model if participants deemed it both unimportant and infrequently performed (as indicated by a composite score of less than 3.0).

All 246 Sub-competencies met the 3.0 threshold when the data were aggregated across work settings. To explore whether the Competencies were truly "generic," the PES experts suggested the use of an additional criterion for including Sub-competencies in the model. Specifically, PES recommended that a generic Sub-competency could be defined (through the mean composite scores) as one that is important and frequently practiced in the majority of work settings. The HEJA 2010-TF readily recognized the utility of this criterion in light of the intended use of the model for professional preparation, certification, and professional development efforts. Though there was a potential risk of losing Sub-competencies specific to a particular work setting, the task force chose the greater benefit of establishing a model that would be representative of the majority of health education specialists. Extensive deliberation resulted in the decision to define a generic Sub-competency as one whose mean composite score met the threshold of 3.0 in at least five of the seven designated practice settings (excluding "other," see Table 2.2). Four of the 246 Sub-competencies, all from the research-related Area of Responsibility used in the survey, failed to meet this threshold for inclusion and were dropped from the model:

- *Assess the feasibility of conducting research*
- *Create a logic model to guide research*
- *Analyze data using inferential and/or other advanced statistical techniques*
- *Disseminate research findings through professional journal publications*

Entry- and advanced-level Sub-competencies

The 242 generic Sub-competencies included in the model were analyzed to identify differences between entry-level and advanced-level Sub-competencies. The HEJA 2010-TF determined that a combination of educational degree and experience level would be most useful to explore potential differences between levels of practice. Accordingly, subgroups of survey respondents were created: bachelor degree with fewer than five years of experience, master's degree with fewer than five years of experience, bachelor degree with five or more years of experience, master's degree with five or more years of experience, and doctoral degree with five of more years of experience. Pairwise comparisons were conducted comparing the composite scores among the five subgroups for each Sub-competency. The Bonferroni correction was used to control for Type 1 error (Tabachnick & Fidell, 2005).

The HEJA 2010-TF then examined patterns of statistically significant differences between the subgroups to identify Sub-competencies that were practiced more frequently or were considered more important by advanced-level health education specialists, as indicated by statistically significantly higher composite scores. Through a series of decision-making steps, 61 of the 242 Sub-competencies were classified as advanced-level only and the remaining 176 Sub-competencies were included as both entry- and advanced-level competencies. For the sake of convenience, the term "entry-level" is used to refer to these 176 Sub-competencies although these Sub-competencies are also practiced and included in the model at the advanced-levels. The distinction between the entry- and advanced-levels of the model is that the *advanced-levels* also include the additional 61 advanced-level only Sub-competencies.

The task force concluded its model development work with the creation of a model containing entry-level and advanced-level Sub-competencies. It recommended that the HEJA 2010-SC continue to explore the advanced Sub-competencies with the goal of determining if the two distinct levels of advanced Sub-competencies could be distinguished. Accordingly, the sponsoring organizations authorized additional analyses designed to isolate and further analyze the subset of 61 Sub-competencies previously validated as *advanced-level only* to determine whether any of these Sub-competencies should be categorized as advanced 1 or advanced 2 Sub-competencies. As in previous analyses, the composite scores of the respondents were compared, which combined frequency and weighted importance ratings into a single data point. Based on the definition of the advanced 2-level developed in the CUP study (five or more years of experience and a doctoral degree), the composite scores of the 133 respondents who met this experience- and degree-based definition were compared to the composite scores of the 647 respondents with five or more years of experience but with less than a doctoral degree (those with bachelor/master's degrees). Statistical significance testing was performed using repeated pairwise comparisons between the composite scores from each subgroup for each Sub-competency. These comparisons yielded numerous statistically significant differences between the combined Baccalaureate/Master's subgroup and the PhD subgroup. In total, 19 of the 61 *advanced-level only* Sub-competencies were identified as advanced 2-level competencies with the remaining 42 of the 61 designated as advanced 1-level Sub-competencies.

Model refinement

As stated earlier in this report, the HEJA 2010-TF decided to use the opportunity afforded by this job analysis to address a frequently-arising question in the profession about Competency-related differences and similarities between evaluation and research. To explore this topic, the task force created two separate survey sections, each of which contained Sub-competencies specifically designated as either research or evaluation. Some Sub-competencies in these two sections were "nearly identical" in that the wording of the Sub-competency was the same with the exception of the context in which it was performed (e.g., *Assess feasibility of conducting evaluation and Assess feasibility of conducting research*). Other Sub-competencies were considered more specific to only one of the survey sections (e.g., *Disseminate research findings through professional conference presentations* had no equivalent in the evaluation content). For purposes of the survey, evaluation was defined as the assessment of the quality and effectiveness of health education programs and/or interventions for the purpose of improvement, and research was defined as the systematic investigation of the relationships between health and health-related factors, the results of which may be generalized to other settings or populations.

As previously stated all of the Sub-competencies in the evaluation section of the survey, and all but four of the Sub-competencies in the research section, were identified as generic to the majority of work settings and were included in the model. Considerations for recombining research and evaluation into a single Area of Responsibility included the benefits of streamlining the overall size of the model, combining nearly identical Sub-competencies that differed only by the context in which they were performed, and avoiding an over-emphasis on Sub-competencies specific to research that tended to be more highly rated in importance by advanced 2-level participants than participants at other levels; however, a challenge to recombining the two Areas lay in detected distinctions in the entry versus advanced-only classifications for some nearly identical Sub-competencies.

Because overall benefits outweighed the potential challenges, the two Areas were recombined in the resulting model. For nearly identical Sub-competencies for which there were no distinctions between entry-level and advanced-level practice, the Sub-competencies were recombined. Nearly identical Sub-competencies for which these entry- and advanced-level distinctions were evident were kept separate and included in the model at appropriate levels. The process resulted in a reduction of total Sub-competencies from 242 to 223.

The validated model

A model of the practice of health education was updated, refined and validated through the HEJA 2010 process. The HEJA 2010 Model consists of 223 Sub-competencies organized into 34 Competencies within the following Seven Areas of Responsibility:

I. Assess needs, assets, and capacity for health education
II. Plan health education
III. Implement health education
IV. Conduct evaluation and research related to health education
V. Administer and manage health education
VI. Serve as a health education resource person
VII. Communicate and advocate for health and health education

The three distinct levels of practice established through the CUP study (NCHEC, SOPHE, & AAHE, 2006) were verified in this study. These three levels were identified as entry (less than five years of experience and a baccalaureate or master's degree), advanced 1 (five or more years of experience and a baccalaureate or master's degree), and advanced 2 (five or more years of experience and a doctoral degree). Consistent with CUP findings, these practice levels represent a hierarchical model in which the two advanced-levels include Sub-competencies used at entry-level, along with additional *advanced-only* Sub-competencies. Of the 223 Sub-competencies identified in the study, 61 were validated as advanced-level only (42 advanced 1 and 19 advanced 2 Sub-competencies). These Sub-competencies are organized within 34 Competencies in seven major Areas of Responsibility. Specific numbers of Competencies and Sub-competencies for each Area of Responsibility are listed below. More details about the model are provided in Section III.

Area I: 7 Competencies – 40 Sub-competencies
  • 34 entry-level
  • 2 advanced 1-level
  • 4 advanced 2-level
Area II: 5 Competencies – 29 Sub-competencies
  • 21 entry-level
  • 6 advanced 1-level
  • 2 advanced 2-level
Area III: 3 Competencies – 20 Sub-competencies
  • 15 entry-level
  • 5 advanced 1-level
Area IV: 5 Competencies – 34 Sub-competencies
  • 25 entry-level
  • 9 advanced 2-level
Area V: 5 Competencies – 37 Sub-competencies
  • 19 entry-level
  • 18 advanced 1-level
Area VI: 3 Competencies – 23 Sub-competencies
  • 12 entry-level
  • 11 advanced 1-level
Area VII: 6 Competencies – 40 Sub-competencies
  • 36 entry-level
  • 4 advanced 2-level

Validated knowledge items

A newly generated list of 113 validated knowledge items emerged from this study. These items, ranked in terms of levels of cognitive usage based on the Revised Bloom's Taxonomy (Anderson & Krathwohl, 2001), were used by at least 50% of study participants. Example knowledge areas include theory, community organization, professional ethics, advocacy, and policy development. A list of these knowledge items and an overview of recommendations for their use is included in Section VI.

Discussion

Interpretation of HEJA 2010 outcomes should be considered within the context of some study limitations. As in previous research, lack of any one comprehensive database of health education specialists made identifying health education specialists in all practice settings a challenge. Though the national CHES database accessed through NCHEC was a valuable and reliable source for sampling CHES, access to potential non-CHES participants was limited to voluntary responses to invitations issued through professional organiza-tions. This access challenge was also an issue in the CUP study (NCHEC, SOPHE, & AAHE, 2006) in which extensive efforts to access and recruit participants through membership lists and other means resulted in "…too few respondents from the business/industry work setting for any meaningful analysis and no respondents in the university health service category" (p. 15). Though some representation of these two work settings was evident in the HEJA 2010 study, the group percentages of each in relation to the total sample, as well as the group percentage for participants working in a school setting, were relatively small. Finding ways to address this ongoing challenge of access to the profession for future job analyses should be a priority.

A second area in which potential limitations should be discussed lies in the use of an online format and four-week window for survey completion. Use of an e-mail-based survey was recommended by PES experts who follow industry guidelines and standards for analysis methodologies and recommendations for periodic updates (every five-seven years); however, this approach limited participation to those who had access to the Internet and were able and inclined to complete the survey within the specified time frame. The 21.5% response rate in this study was comparable to that obtained in other job analyses conducted by PES, and is in line with the range of response rates generally found in professional job analyses. Given that the average amount of time required to complete the survey was close to one hour, the responses obtained were considered a reflection of the opinions of a cohort of thoughtful and committed health education specialists.

It should also be noted that the multi-phasic process of developing the 246 Sub-competencies used in the HEJA 2010 survey was, in itself, a research-valid part of the analysis. The 59 volunteer health education specialists who participated in the instrument-development process were carefully selected from a volunteer pool to represent diverse work settings, geographic regions, levels of experience, and other relevant demographics in the profession. Qualitative focus group and structured interview procedures were used to guide representative subgroups of this sample in the sequential phases of instrument development. A modified Delphi technique was used to involve the HEJA 2010-TF in instrument-shaping decisions at strategic points throughout the process; therefore, it should be no surprise that 242 of the 246 Sub-competencies emerging from the instrument development process were also validated for model inclusion based on actual survey responses. The fact that, once evaluation and research Sub-competencies were re-combined, the resulting 223 Sub-competencies were validated for model inclusion using the same composite score procedures and inclusion criteria as in the CUP study lends further credence to procedure validity.

Despite these indicators of study validity, some revisions to the approach are recommended for future analyses. For example, the decision to bring together volunteers with varying work settings and levels of experience was a valid approach to ensure diverse representation and should be repeated; however, this diversity also generated the need for additional discussions about profession-generic terminology and the basics of competency development. Though the PES experts who guided this process provided the needed context for each task, the development of a written guide for volunteers to use when developing Sub-competency statements, for example, could be useful in expediting the process.

The need to meet the certification industry standard of conducting a job analysis every five-seven years calls for a more extensive, yet efficient, approach to participant sampling. Finding ways to access a wider representation of work settings, and a larger total number of health education specialists, for future job analyses is recommended. The need to provide updated analysis results every five years to maintain the profession's accreditation status will require establishing an ongoing system for periodic updates.

Summary

In summary, the HEJA 2010 study was a multi-phased national study implemented to validate the contemporary practice of entry- and advanced-level health education specialists. The 15 steps illustrated in Figure 2.1 represent the work of 59 volunteer professionals representing the diversity of health education work settings, educational backgrounds, and experience levels of the profession. These volunteers included an eleven-member HEJA 2010 task force and five-member HEJA 2010 steering committee. This task force, with support from the steering committee, worked with the PES experts to complete nearly two years of planning, execution, data analyses, and model development.

The HEJA 2010 outcomes re-affirmed Seven Areas of Responsibility for health education specialists. New and/or expanded Competencies were identified in Areas related to ethics, partnership development, training, consultative relationships, influencing policy, and promoting the health education profession. 113 knowledge items relevant to health education practice were also developed and empirically validated for the first time. A hierarchical model of practice was verified at entry-, advanced 1-, and advanced 2-levels.

More details about the HEJA 2010 Model and knowledge list and recommendations for their use are included in subsequent sections. A comparison of the HEJA 2010 Model and the former CUP Model (NCHEC, SOPHE, & AAHE, 2006) is also provided. ◆

Section III:
The HEJA 2010 Model

Section III: The HEJA 2010 Model

The HEJA 2010 Model (see Table 3.1) contains a common set of Competencies used in the entry- and advanced-level practice of health education specialists. Because these Competencies are generic across work settings, they should serve as the basis for professional preparation, credentialing, and professional development for all health education specialists. It is recommended that the entry-level Competencies and Sub-competencies be addressed in baccalaureate programs and graduate programs (see Section IV) ("Competencies Update Project," 2008, para. 8). Graduate programs should also incorporate the advanced 1- and advanced 2-level Competencies and Sub-competencies.

It is possible that some additional setting-specific Competencies may be warranted in some work settings. For example, those working in community health settings may need more preparation in public health policy; the application of worksite safety regulations may be needed in some corporate settings; and teaching methodologies may be needed for those preparing to teach in schools. Thus, some additional, setting-specific Competencies may be needed in some professional preparation and professional development efforts.

In addition to some wording and content changes, a new numbering system was adopted as a replacement to the former "letters and single numbers" approach. Throughout the HEJA 2010 process, the taskforce and others discovered that references to specific Sub-competencies using the former system of alphabetical letters for Competencies and a single-digit number for Sub-competencies within each Area was sometimes confusing. For example, the letter "A" was used for the first Competency in each Area and the number "1" was used for each Sub-competency in each Competency across all Areas. Though it was feasible to use such labels as "I-A-1" to refer to the first Sub-competency under Competency A in Area I, the need to also use letters to refer to the practice levels of Entry (E), Advanced 1 (A1), and Advanced 2 (A2) rendered a "lettering system" even more confusing. The PES experts and NCHEC board directors who regularly worked with these Sub-competencies to create items for the CHES certification exam used a numbering system that was conceptually easier to use. In this 3-point numbering system, the first number referred to the Area of Responsibility, the second number referred to the Competency within that Area, and the third number referring to the Sub-competency. For example, under Area IV of the model, the second Sub-competency under the first Competency would be 4.1.2. Under Area I, the first Sub-competency under Competency 2 would be 1.2.1.

This numbering system was adopted for the HEJA 2010 Model to simplify, and provide a consistent approach to, the way in which Competencies and Sub-competencies are labeled and used. Though Roman numerals will still be used when referring to the Seven Areas of Responsibility when the areas stand alone, the Arabic numbers will be used for the Areas as part of the numbering system when referring to Competencies and Sub-competencies.

Table 3.1

Health Educator Job Analysis 2010 Model: Overview of Areas of Responsibility and Competencies

Area I: Assess Needs, Assets, and Capacity for Health Education

1.1: Plan assessment process
1.2: Access existing information and data related to health
1.3: Collect quantitative and/or qualitative data related to health
1.4: Examine relationships among behavioral, environmental and genetic factors that enhance or compromise health
1.5: Examine factors that influence the learning process
1.6: Examine factors that enhance or compromise the process of health education
1.7: Infer needs for health education based on assessment findings

Area II: Plan Health Education

2.1: Involve priority populations and other stakeholders in the planning process
2.2: Develop goals and objectives
2.3: Select or design strategies and interventions
2.4: Develop a scope and sequence for the delivery of health education
2.5: Address factors that affect implementation

Area III: Implement Health Education

3.1: Implement a plan of action
3.2: Monitor implementation of health education
3.3: Train individuals involved in implementation of health education

Area IV: Conduct Evaluation and Research Related to Health Education

4.1: Develop evaluation/research plan
4.2: Design instruments to collect evaluation/research data
4.3: Collect and analyze evaluation/research data
4.4: Interpret results of the evaluation/research
4.5: Apply findings from evaluation/research

Area V: Administer and Manage Health Education

5.1: Manage fiscal resources
5.2: Obtain acceptance and support for programs
5.3: Demonstrate leadership
5.4: Manage human resources
5.5: Facilitate partnerships in support of health education

Area VI: Serve as a Health Education Resource Person

6.1: Obtain and disseminate health-related information
6.2: Provide training
6.3: Serve as a health education consultant

Area VII: Communicate and Advocate for Health and Health Education

7.1: Assess and prioritize health information and advocacy needs
7.2: Identify and develop a variety of communication strategies, methods, and techniques
7.3: Deliver messages using a variety of strategies, methods and techniques
7.4: Engage in health education advocacy
7.5: Influence policy to promote health
7.6: Promote the health education profession

Area I: Assess Needs, Assets, and Capacity for Health Education

The role

The primary purpose of a needs assessment is to gather information to determine what health education activities are appropriate in a given setting. Needs may be basic–that is, essential to the comfort and well-being of every human being (food, water, warmth, oxygen, etc.)–or indicators of a gap between conditions as they are and as they ought to be. Although the term "problem" is frequently used interchangeably with "need" in health education, strictly speaking they are different. A health problem is defined as a potential or real threat to physical or emotional well-being.

Needs assessment is the systematic, planned collection of information about the health knowledge, perceptions, attitudes, motivation, and practices of individuals or groups and the quality of the socioeconomic environment in which they live (see Table 3.2). Logically, assessment of needs should precede program planning. This process provides data that determine whether a health education program is justified, and if so, what its nature and emphasis ought to be.

To successfully conduct a needs assessment, it is necessary to identify health-related databases and valid sources of data. It is also necessary to be able to gather data with appropriate instruments, apply survey techniques, and identify behaviors that influence health. Determining the extent of existing services and gaps in the provision of services is critical, along with the ability to analyze data and determine priorities for health education.

Settings

The following text describes how a needs assessment is used in different practice settings.

Community setting. The health education specialist in the community setting relies on many sources of current data, such as health planning agencies, public health departments, census reports, and interviews with community leaders and members of the priority population. Data provide information about perceived health needs. If specific behaviors or health practices are causally linked to the incidence of major health problems, then a health education program may be planned to motivate and facilitate voluntary, desirable changes in those behaviors.

School (K-12) setting. In the school setting, local, state, and national data are used to determine the scope and sequence of curricula and to identify strengths and weaknesses to aid in developing a Coordinated School Health Program. National-level and state-level data may be considered and utilized, but local data are essential to good curriculum planning. Information about health knowledge, attitudes, skills, and practices can be gathered directly from students and used to improve health instruction, school policies, and the school environment. Information gathered from parents, administrators, and school health personnel by a "Healthy School Team," consisting of representatives from each of the eight components of the Coordinated School Health Program, can assist in identifying potential gaps in creating a healthy school community.

Health care setting. In the health care setting, complaints by health professionals about a growing number of emergency room visits, for example, might lead the health education specialist to survey records to determine whether the problem is general or limited to patients with particular kinds of emergencies or with situational needs (e.g., patients without adequate health insurance or with limited access to primary care physicians). An assessment of the reasons for this trend would help to determine what services or policies could help improve the situation.

Business/industry setting. In the workplace, a health education specialist might work with medical professionals to analyze data that can be used to identify health needs of the workers, for example, data about health insurance claims, absenteeism and its causes, types of accidents and severity of injuries, and compensation claims. In addition, a health education specialist in this setting should survey employees to discover their felt needs and interests. Analysis of these data would indicate priority needs for health promotion programs.

College/university setting. In the college or university setting, health education specialists are often involved in assessing student performance in meeting state and national standards in order to maintain accreditation. Tracking students' progress in meeting the standards, assessing the learning environment, and linking the two are important for revising the curriculum and meeting accreditation requirements.

University health services setting. The health education specialist who practices in student health services works side-by-side with clinical practitioners. The health education specialist assesses the health needs of students, staff, and faculty through the use of focus groups, surveys, and interviews. In the assessment process, it is important to develop avenues for obtaining information on perceptions, attitudes, practices, and felt needs in addition to health problems and practices.

Table 3.2
Health Educator Job Analysis 2010 Model: Area I: Assess needs, assets, and capacity for health education

SECTION: III

Competency	Entry	Advanced 1	Advanced 2
1.1 Plan assessment process	1.1.1 Identify existing and needed resources to conduct assessments 1.1.3 Apply theories and models to develop assessment strategies 1.1.4 Develop plans for data collection, analysis, and interpretation 1.1.6 Integrate research designs, methods, and instruments into assessment plans	1.1.2 Identify stakeholders to participate in the assessment process 1.1.5 Engage stakeholders to participate in the assessment process	
1.2 Access existing information and data related to health	1.2.1 Identify sources of data related to health 1.2.2 Critique sources of health information using theory and evidence from the literature 1.2.3 Select valid sources of information about health 1.2.4 Identify gaps in data using theories and assessment models 1.2.5 Establish collaborative relationships and agreements that facilitate access to data 1.2.6 Conduct searches of existing databases for specific health-related data		
1.3 Collect quantitative and/or qualitative data related to health	1.3.1 Collect primary and/or secondary data 1.3.2 Integrate primary data with secondary data 1.3.3 Identify data collection instruments and methods 1.3.4 Develop data collection instruments and methods 1.3.5 Train personnel and stakeholders regarding data collection 1.3.6 Use data collection instruments and methods 1.3 7 Employ ethical standards when collecting data		

Competency	Entry	Advanced 1	Advanced 2
1.4 Examine relationships among behavioral, environmental and genetic factors that enhance or compromise health	1.4.1 Identify factors that influence health behaviors 1.4.2 Analyze factors that influence health behaviors 1.4.3 Identify factors that enhance or compromise health 1.4.4 Analyze factors that enhance or compromise health		
1.5 Examine factors that influence the learning process	1.5 1 Identify factors that foster or hinder the learning process 1.5 3 Identify factors that foster or hinder attitudes and beliefs 1.5 4 Analyze factors that foster or hinder attitudes and beliefs		1.5.2 Analyze factors that foster or hinder the learning process 1.5.5 Identify factors that foster or hinder skill building 1.5.6 Analyze factors that foster or hinder skill building
1.6 Examine factors that enhance or compromise the process of health education	1.6.1 Determine the extent of available health education programs, interventions, and policies 1.6.2 Assess the quality of available health education programs, interventions, and policies 1.6.3 Identify existing and potential partners for the provision of health education 1.6.4 Assess social, environmental, and political conditions that may impact health education 1.6.5 Analyze the capacity for developing needed health education 1.6.6 Assess the need for resources to foster health education		
1.7 Infer needs for health education based on assessment findings	1.7.1 Analyze assessment findings 1.7.3 Prioritize health education needs 1.7.4 Identify emerging health education needs 1.7.5 Report assessment findings		1.7.2 Synthesize assessment findings

SECTION: III

Area II: Plan Health Education

The role.

Program planning begins with the assessment of existing health needs, problems, and concerns (see Table 3.3). The extent to which these are directly linked to health behaviors determines the specific changes in behaviors for which the program planning process is set in motion. Relevant people are identified and involved in the project, objectives are established, educational methods are selected, and resources are located. It is within this process that planning for program evaluation begins as well.

Settings.

The following text describes how planning is used in different practice settings:

Community setting. In a community setting where a needs assessment has identified a significant health problem, the health education specialist convenes representatives of relevant groups to identify populations in need of health education. The health education specialist also seeks input and promotes involvement from those who will affect and be affected by the program. Health education specialists should rely on the results of the needs assessment and available research to apply principles of community organization to integrate health education within existing health programs. Another key Responsibility of health education specialists is to formulate objectives and develop interventions appropriate to meet the needs of target populations. Identifying and assessing community resources and barriers affecting implementation of the program unique to the community setting can help health education specialists achieve this. The selection of program activities and interventions depends on the characteristics of the priority population, its constraints and concerns, the budget and timeframe, and the fit between program schedules and other obligations of the participants.

School (K-12) setting. The decision to provide health education in schools is usually made by administrators or mandated by policy or law. The school health education specialist organizes an advisory committee (consisting of teachers, administrators, members of the community, representatives from voluntary agencies, parents, youth group leaders, clergy, and students) to select or develop health education curricula and materials. These decisions should be based on research results and best practices and should consider available resources and barriers to implementation, such as time and space. Objectives should be based on the needs of school-aged children and adolescents. Curricula should follow a logical scope and sequence.

Health care setting. The health education specialist in the health care setting works with nurses, physicians, nutritionists, physical therapists, and other health care professionals to plan patient and community education programs. The team develops education programs for patients and their families to promote compliance with medical directions and enhance understanding of medical procedures and conditions. The role of the health education specialist in this setting is to assist the team in establishing objectives, identifying staff roles in providing education, selecting teaching methods and strategies, evaluating results, documenting the education effort, designing promotion activities, and training interdisciplinary staff to conduct the program, as appropriate.

Business/industry setting. In the workplace, the health education specialist analyzes data from numerous sources (including insurance records, safety records, workers' compensation claims, and employee self-report questionnaires) to provide a basis for a presentation to management outlining the benefits and costs of a health education program. After gaining administrative support, the health education specialist convenes an employee committee with representatives from all levels of the organization to make recommendations concerning program priorities, objectives, scheduling, publicity, incentives, and fees. The health education specialist leads the team in developing data- and theory-based interventions and strategies to meet the needs of employees.

College/university setting. The health education specialist in a higher education setting analyzes research results, current professional competencies, accreditation standards, and certification requirements and uses the results to design professional preparation programs that will encourage the development of essential health education planning competencies in candidates, regardless of future practice setting.

University health services setting. The health education specialist who practices in student health services works side by side with clinical practitioners. The health education specialist uses the needs assessment to develop program and behavioral objectives and to design interventions that reduce health risks and improve health. The health education specialist works with clinical practitioners and others to integrate health education into other programs, including treatment regimens and campus-wide activities. The health education specialist also evaluates the efficacy of educational methods in achieving objectives.

Table 3.3
Health Educator Job Analysis 2010 Model: Area II: Plan health education

Competency	Entry	Advanced 1	Advanced 2
2.1 Involve priority populations and other stakeholders in the planning process	2.1.1 Incorporate principles of community organization 2.1.2 Identify priority populations and other stakeholders 2.1.3 Communicate need for health education to priority populations and other stakeholders 2.1.4 Develop collaborative efforts among priority populations and other stakeholders 2.1.5 Elicit input from priority populations and other stakeholders 2.1.6 Obtain commitments from priority populations and other stakeholders		
2.2 Develop goals and objectives	2.2.2 Identify desired outcomes utilizing the needs assessment results 2.2.6 Assess resources needed to achieve objectives	2.2.1 Use assessment results to inform the planning process 2.2.4 Develop goal statements 2.2.5 Formulate specific, measurable, attainable, realistic, and time-sensitive objectives	2.2.3 Select planning model(s) for health education
2.3 Select or design strategies and interventions	2.3.2 Design theory-based strategies and interventions to achieve stated objectives 2.3.4 Comply with legal and ethical principles in designing strategies and interventions 2.3.5 Apply principles of cultural competence in selecting and designing strategies and interventions 2.3.6 Pilot test strategies and interventions	2.3.3 Select a variety of strategies and interventions to achieve stated objectives	2.3.1 Assess efficacy of various strategies to ensure consistency with objectives

Competency	Entry	Advanced 1	Advanced 2
2.4 Develop a scope and sequence for the delivery of health education	2.4.1 Determine the range of health education needed to achieve goals and objectives 2.4.2 Select resources required to implement health education 2.4.3 Use logic models to guide the planning process 2.4.6 Analyze the opportunity for integrating health education into other programs 2.4.7 Develop a process for integrating health education into other programs	2.4.4 Organize health education into a logical sequence 2.4.5 Develop a timeline for the delivery of health education	
2.5 Address factors that affect implementation	2.5.1 Identify factors that foster or hinder implementation 2.5.2 Analyze factors that foster or hinder implementation 2.5.3 Use findings of pilot to refine implementation plans as needed 2.5.4 Develop a conducive learning environment		

Area III: Implement Health Education

The role.

Health education specialists educate and motivate people in their pursuit of healthful behaviors. Regardless of the setting in which they work, health education specialists must be able to infer objectives suitable to the program, select media and methods appropriate to the intended audience, conduct programs as planned, make revisions to programs and objectives, and train those involved in implementation of the program, all consistent with results from having monitored their programs in action (see Table 3.4).

Settings.

The following text describes how implementation is used in different practice settings:

Community setting. Health education specialists working for behavior change in the community face dual challenges of motivating a diverse population to pursue healthful behaviors. Health education specialists may also desire to change the community environment, norms or capacity. Therefore, health education specialists working in the community setting must use a variety of coordinated approaches to reach program objectives. A health education specialist attempting to improve families' dietary choices, for example, might form an advisory group or community coalition to ensure community needs, interests, and cultures are incorporated into the program. He or she would identify a wide range of intervention strategies to be carried out in a number of locations in order to engage sub-groups of the population. Examples of such intervention strategies include increasing awareness of dietary choices through local media, coordinating with local grocery chains to provide educational materials and stock healthier items, arranging for a cooking demonstration at a community center or other place of gathering for the intended audiences, collaborating with community planners to make a community vegetable garden or farmer's market available, or working with schools to change vending machine policies.

School (K-12) setting. In the school setting, health education specialists work to increase students' knowledge and to promote positive attitudes and behaviors with respect to health. Typically provided with a curriculum by the school administration, a school-based health education specialist infers objectives appropriate to students' learning potential and abilities and decides on appropriate teaching techniques. Lesson plans are informed by the health education specialist's awareness of the students' learning needs, degree of parental support, and related factors. Student learning is assessed and monitored to facilitate revisions in the curriculum and instructional methods. The health education specialist also works with administrative staff, faculty, parent groups and community groups to encourage school policies that support healthy behaviors.

Health care setting. Health education specialists employed in health care settings function as independent participants, as well as liaisons between patients and providers. A health education specialist in this setting might conduct a program to support patients' weight loss efforts. He or she might offer classes, supported by presentations from the health care providers, and make use of educational materials consistent with the patients' needs. The health education specialist might arrange for opportunities to apply the information learned through cooking classes or a grocery store tour to improve ability to read food labels. He or she would monitor participant outcomes and providers' reactions, the process of delivering such activities, and would make changes to the program and objectives as warranted.

Business/industry setting. In the workplace, health education specialists work with employers to offer educational programs that respond to employees' health needs (such as programs to improve diet) in a manner conducive to employee participation. The health education specialist would need to understand the needs and interests of employees, as well as the workplace culture and ways of doing business that might affect healthy behaviors. Employees might be offered healthful food choices in the company cafeteria, exercise classes, stress reduction counseling, and smoking cessation therapy, all supplemented by educational materials.

College/university setting. A health education specialist working in a higher education setting might conduct an introductory-level health class in which he or she guides each student through a personal change project tailored to the student's interests, preparedness for the course, and learning style. Objectives of the project would be determined and modified as required to fit the needs of the student and the class. Instructional methods such as PowerPoint presentations, use of technology, and role-playing might be used.

Student feedback and instructor observations can be used to refine future programs to more effectively achieve goals within a course's curriculum.

University health services setting. In conjunction with health care providers, health education specialists in a university health services setting work with the entire university community. Programs are constructed in response to established needs of faculty, staff, and students. For example, with the support of appropriate university personnel, the health education specialist might work with residence hall officials to offer educational sessions in student dormitories on contraception, alcohol use, or dating violence. Program availability would match student needs and be supported by media intended to appeal to the college student. Incentives could be offered to encourage attendance. The health education specialist would monitor students' interest and attendance and request feedback from students and instructors to improve future programs.

Table 3.4

Health Educator Job Analysis 2010 Model: Area III: Implement health education

Competency	Entry	Advanced 1	Advanced 2
3.1 Implement a plan of action	3.1.1 Assess readiness for implementation 3.1.2 Collect baseline data 3.1.3 Use strategies to ensure cultural competence in implementing health education plans 3.1.4 Use a variety of strategies to deliver a plan of action 3.1.5 Promote plan of action 3.1.6 Apply theories and models of implementation 3.1.7 Launch plan of action		
3.2 Monitor implementation of health education	3.2.1 Monitor progress in accordance with timeline 3.2.2 Assess progress in achieving objectives 3.2.3 Modify plan of action as needed 3.2.4 Monitor use of resources 3.2.5 Monitor compliance with legal and ethical principles		
3.3 Train individuals involved in implementation of health education	3.3.1 Select training participants needed for implementation 3.3.5 Demonstrate a wide range of training strategies 3.3.6 Deliver training	3.3.2 Identify training needs 3.3.3 Develop training objectives 3.3.4 Create training using best practices 3.3.7 Evaluate training 3.3.8 Use evaluation findings to plan future training	

Area IV: Conduct Evaluation and Research Related to Health Education

The role.

Health education specialists at all levels are expected to be able to conduct a thorough review of the literature and to apply research findings from basic and evaluative research (see Table 3.5). They may also be expected to conduct evaluations of policy, projects, and programs. The ability to aggregate data from one or more programs for the purpose of establishing a point of reference and making comparisons is also important. As the health education specialist progresses within the profession, the required level of skill in conducting research and evaluation becomes more advanced. Health education specialists may be expected to write applications for funding, including research proposals. The ability to evaluate a policy or a program's effectiveness is essential to maintaining its support and funding in an increasingly competitive environment.

Advanced-level health education specialists should be able to: draw on various measures to establish the economic impact of health education and health promotion programs; help identify other professionals needed for collaborative approaches; and provide information to governments, employers, and program funding sources. They should be able to translate research findings into lay language, making health communications more credible.

Settings.

The following text describes how evaluation is used in different practice settings:

Community setting. The health education specialist may use epidemiological principles to explain disease outbreaks or define high-risk neighborhoods within communities that require special program emphasis. The discussion of any topic important to the community, such as unintentional injuries, an outbreak of measles or food poisoning, or sexually transmitted infections requires mastery of research principles and language. Evaluations may provide necessary information to support programs when reviewed by local or state governments. Competitive proposals not only help secure funding, but also may further encourage collaborative projects within a community.

School (K-12) setting. Health education specialists practicing in the school setting may be called upon to assist in the documentation of student health knowledge, attitudes and behaviors. Data gained from a review of the literature and from qualitative and quantitative research are provided by health education specialists to school boards and parents in order to help them understand students' needs and interests. Evaluation of goals, objectives, and learning activities is critical to identifying, selecting, and implementing effective curricula. As accountability grows, both qualitative and quantitative research methods are increasingly being emphasized in school settings.

Health care setting. A health education specialist practicing in a health care setting must be able to understand and interpret research findings for patients and their families, and may be asked to participate as a member of a research team that investigates behavioral components of adherence to clinical regimens. As medical technologies and treatments are advanced through the conduct of clinical trials, evaluative research becomes increasingly important in addressing chronic disease conditions and the reduction of health-risk behaviors for primary prevention.

Business/industry setting. Adults spend the majority of their time in the workplace. Health education specialists in this setting need qualitative and quantitative research skills to demonstrate the efficacy of worksite health promotion programs and the contributions of such programs to productivity and organizational goals. Health education specialists may also be asked to assist in monitoring the work environment for safety compliance and injury reduction. Additionally, using evaluative research, health education specialists may be able to help determine quality and cost-effectiveness of competing health plans to benefit employers and employees.

College/university setting. Health education specialists are expected to engage in scholarly endeavors that include research, grant writing, and dissemination of research findings. In addition to instructional and administrative responsibilities, university health education specialists frequently collaborate with others within and outside of their respective institutions. These efforts contribute to the scientific body of knowledge encompassing health behavior, disease prevention, and risk reduction strategies and to the discipline of health education.

University health services setting. Health education specialists working in the university health services setting face many of the same issues as those in the business/industry and health care settings. These health education specialists need skills in all facets of research including qualitative and quantitative research. Skills in evaluative research are necessary to determine the efficacy and cost-effectiveness of programs for university faculty, staff, and students.

Table 3.5
Health Educator Job Analysis 2010 Model: Area IV: Conduct evaluation and research related to health education

Competency	Entry	Advanced 1	Advanced 2
4.1 Develop evaluation/ research plan	4.1.3 Assess feasibility of conducting evaluation/ research 4.1.4 Critique evaluation and research methods and findings found in the related literature 4.1.5 Synthesize information found in the literature 4.1.6 Assess the merits and limitations of qualitative and quantitative data collection for evaluation 4.1.8 Identify existing data collection instruments 4.1.9 Critique existing data collection instruments for evaluation 4.1.12 Develop data analysis plan for evaluation 4.1.14 Apply ethical standards in developing the evaluation/ research plan		4.1.1 Create purpose statement 4.1.2 Develop evaluation/ research questions 4.1.7 Assess the merits and limitations of qualitative and quantitative data collection for research 4.1.10 Critique existing data collection instruments for research 4.1.11 Create a logic model to guide the evaluation process 4.1.13 Develop data analysis plan for research
4.2 Design instruments to collect evaluation/ research data	4.2.1 Identify useable questions from existing instruments 4.2.2 Write new items to be used in data collection for evaluation 4.2.4 Establish validity of data collection instruments 4.2.5 Establish reliability of data collection instruments		4.2.3 Write new items to be used in data collection for research
4.3 Collect and analyze evaluation/ research data	4.3.1 Collect data based on the evaluation/research plan 4.3.2 Monitor data collection and management 4.3.3 Analyze data using descriptive statistics 4.3.4 Analyze data using inferential and/or other advanced statistical methods 4.3.5 Analyze data using qualitative methods 4.3.6 Apply ethical standards in collecting and analyzing data		

Competency	Entry	Advanced 1	Advanced 2
4.4 Interpret results of the evaluation/ research	4.4.1 Compare results to evaluation/research questions 4.4.2 Compare results to other findings 4.4.3 Propose possible explanations of findings 4.4.4 Identify possible limitations of findings 4.4.5 Develop recommendations based on results		
4.5 Apply findings from evaluation/ research	4.5.1 Communicate findings to stakeholders 4.5.3 Apply findings in policy analysis and program development		4.5.2 Evaluate feasibility of implementing recommendations from evaluation 4.5.4 Disseminate research findings through professional conference presentations

Area V: Administer and Manage Health Education

The role.

Health education specialists are broadly trained to work as systems thinkers with individuals, groups, and communities, and as a result, they can effectively function in multiple roles within the larger context of their institutions or other environments (see Table 3.6). The boundaries between the entry- and advanced-levels become permeable when communities, groups, or organizations have roles to fill and few individuals are well-trained and credentialed.

While some administrative functions may fall to the entry-level health education specialist, administration is generally a function of the more advanced-level individual. Health education specialists often become program managers or supervisors of other health education specialists or teams of allied health professionals. Good management incorporates effective leadership skills with managing fiscal resources, task assignments, and performance evaluation. Supervisors obtain acceptance and support for programs from stakeholders such as higher-level management or staff. This role requires effective communication skills, organizational knowledge, and objectivity. Because of their broad training and their understanding of individuals and communities, health education specialists can be effective managers who consider potential partnerships in the larger context of their institution or environment.

Settings.

The following text describes how administering programs is used in different practice settings:

Community setting. Health education specialists in a community setting may be responsible for managing a program involving several health education specialists and outreach workers who provide programs and explain health agency initiatives. Advanced-level health education specialists may find themselves providing support for or aligning organizational structure with multiple divisions of their local public health departments, such as mental health services, environmental health services, or health planning efforts.

School (K-12) setting. In addition to managing students in the classroom, health education specialists in the school setting find themselves identifying and securing fiscal resources to support coordinated school health programs. Serving as curriculum coordinators or project directors, health education specialists may manage curricular and budgetary issues for the school health program, and may work with school health advisory councils in obtaining acceptance and support for content areas to be addressed in the curriculum. A frequent responsibility of the practicing health education specialist is the supervision of pre-service interns (student teachers). As curriculum specialists or program heads, health education specialists serve as team leaders to promote comprehensive health education in their school, throughout the school district, and at the state level.

Health care settings. Health education specialists may be the managers of professional development programs in major medical complexes, nursing homes, or transitional facilities. The ability to communicate and facilitate partnerships with a variety of medical professionals, aides, volunteers, clients and family, or community members is very important in this setting. Planning programs that contribute to institutional maintenance of accreditation and compliance with government regulations may also be the task of the health education specialist, who may supervise institutional service learning activities that augment staff efforts.

Business/industry setting. In this setting, a health education specialist may lead or be part of a team as a coordinator for an employee assistance program or director of a multi-staff health promotion effort. As an employee, a health education specialist may also supervise or provide support for employed staff, contracted staff, or volunteers in health promotion programs (e.g., smoking cessation, stress management, substance misuse, and weight loss).

College/university setting. Health education specialists in the college/university setting may be involved in a variety of administrative responsibilities, including coordination of professional preparation programs and chairing of an academic department. In this role, the health education specialists must develop and manage the program budgets. Professional preparation programs also have to align their program goals with the college/university's mission and goals. Other Responsibilities might include coordinating and supervising student internships, analyzing the program's curriculum for appropriate goals and objectives, and chairing or facilitating committees.

University health services setting. Health education specialists in the university health services setting may coordinate special campus events, develop campus health initiatives, arrange for campus screenings by other agencies, or develop health education programs for priority populations within the university community. Health education specialists in the college or university setting may also administer health education/promotion programs, or in some cases, the health services center itself. In this role, they must be able to plan, organize the center, administer personnel, secure funds, and manage fiscal resources.

Table 3.6

Health Educator Job Analysis 2010 Model: Area V: Administer and manage health education

Competency	Entry	Advanced 1	Advanced 2
5.1 Manage fiscal resources		5.1.1 Identify fiscal and other resources 5.1.2 Prepare requests/ proposals to obtain fiscal resources 5.1.3 Develop budgets to support health educa-tion efforts 5.1.4 Manage program budgets 5.1.5 Prepare budget reports 5.1.6 Demonstrate ethical behavior in managing fiscal resources	

Competency	Entry	Advanced 1	Advanced 2
5.2 Obtain acceptance and support for programs	5.2.5 Provide support for individuals who deliver professional development opportunities 5.2.6 Explain how program goals align with organizational structure, mission, and goals	5.2.1 Use commu-nication strategies to obtain program support 5.2.2 Facilitate cooperation among stakeholders responsible for health education 5.2.3 Prepare reports to obtain and/or maintain program support 5.2.4 Synthesize data for purposes of reporting	
5.3 Demonstrate leadership	5.3.1 Conduct strategic planning 5.3.2 Analyze an organization's culture in relationship to health education goals 5.3.4 Develop strategies to reinforce or change organi-zational culture to achieve health education goals 5.3.5 Comply with existing laws and regulations 5.3.6 Adhere to ethical standards of the profession 5.3.7 Facilitate efforts to achieve organizational mission 5.3.8 Analyze the need for a systems approach to change 5.3.9 Facilitate needed changes to organizational cultures	5.3.3 Promote collaboration among stakeholders	

Competency	Entry	Advanced 1	Advanced 2
5.4 Manage human resources	5.4.1 Develop volunteer opportunities 5.4.2 Demonstrate leadership skills in managing human resources 5.4.3 Apply human resource policies consistent with relevant laws and regulations 5.4.4 Evaluate qualifications of staff and volunteers needed for programs 5.4.5 Recruit volunteers and staff 5.4.7 Apply appropriate methods for team development 5.4.8 Model professional practices and ethical behavior 5.4.11 Evaluate performance of staff and volunteers	5.4.6 Employ conflict resolution strategies 5.4.9 Develop strategies to enhance staff and volunteers' career development 5.4.10 Implement strategies to enhance staff and volunteers' career development	
5.5 Facilitate partnerships in support of health education	5.5.3 Facilitate partner relationship(s)	5.5.1 Identify potential partner(s) 5.5.2 Assess capacity of potential partner(s) to meet program goals 5.5.4 Elicit feedback from partner(s) 5.5.5 Evaluate feasibility of continuing partnership	

Area VI: Serve as a Health Education Resource Person

The role.

The setting in which the health education specialist functions largely determines the nature of the resources provided. When requested, health education specialists need to serve as a resource for valid and reliable health information and materials (see Table 3.7). They must be: aware of a variety of community resources at the local, state, and national levels; familiar with computer-based retrieval systems and national online databases; and skillful at locating valid information through Internet searches. In addition, the health education specialist needs to be able to evaluate and select appropriate resource materials for dissemination to individuals and groups. Being a resource person also means that the health education specialist must be able to establish consultative relationships and develop the skills necessary for serving as a liaison for networking and for facilitating collaborative efforts.

Settings.

The following text describes how acting as a resource is used in different practice settings:

Community setting. Community settings may include work with community-based organizations, local voluntary health organizations, churches, civic organizations, neighborhood associations, and other non-profits. In the community setting, health education specialists might be asked to serve on various community-wide coalitions to help identify and implement strategies to improve health. Health education specialists can serve as a resource and link to current health related data (e.g., Behavioral Risk Factor Surveillance System, Youth Risk Behavior Surveillance System), research studies, and published best practices in health promotion and disease prevention. In addition, health education specialists can provide suggestions about related sources such as audiovisual materials, educational pamphlets, and posters for distribution.

School (K-12) setting. A health education specialist in the school setting might work with a curriculum committee to identify and select educational materials that comply with state legislative mandates and school district policies. The health education specialist might be asked to provide expert assistance to committee members in examining state laws and codes, establishing criteria for the evaluation of instructional materials, and recommending placement of the topic in the overall curriculum scope and sequence plan. After selection of the material, the health education specialist might also arrange preview sessions for interested parents and community members.

Health care setting. Health care settings may include hospitals, clinics, medical centers, and satellite health clinics. A health education specialist in the health care setting might serve as a consultant to a community group in developing chronic disease prevention and control education programs. The health education specialist would provide information on successful or evidence-based programs, help identify culturally and linguistically appropriate materials, conduct focus groups to assist in planning interventions, identify expert speakers, and help identify media and other communication channels for disseminating information about the program to the community.

Business/industry setting. Physical fitness and nutrition programs are frequently featured in worksite health promotion programming. As a resource person, the health education specialist would be responsible for disseminating information to employers and employees about the program in a timely manner. Health education specialists can identify and organize resources needed for the implementation and continuation of the fitness or other health promotion programs and policy changes at the worksite to promote health. They can identify research data to present to concerned personnel and monitor the plans of those responsible for conducting the program to ensure that its activities match the stated goals and objectives. They can also find relevant posters and brochures about healthy eating and physical activity to display in break rooms and distribute to employees.

College/university setting. The professor or instructor teaching a course in a health education professional preparation program might have students serve as consultants to a local school district to help district team members assess their coordinated school health program using the CDC's School Health Index. As the students work with the local district, they are sharpening their consulting and networking skills, as well as conveying health-related information to key stakeholders in the schools.

University health services setting. The health education specialist in the university health services setting might establish a Web site where students and staff can obtain information about health-related topics, such as nutrition; alcohol, tobacco and other drugs; sexuality; stress reduction; and physical activity. The Web site should contain links to a number of sites containing current and reliable health information.

Table 3.7

Health Educator Job Analysis 2010 Model: Area VI: Serve as a health education resource person

Competency	Entry	Advanced 1	Advanced 2
6.1 Obtain and disseminate health-related information	6.1.1 Assess information needs 6.1.2 Identify valid information resources 6.1.3 Critique resource materials for accuracy, relevance, and timeliness 6.1.4 Convey health-related information to priority populations 6.1.5 Convey health-related information to key stakeholders		
6.2 Provide training	6.2.3 Identify priority populations	6.2.1 Analyze requests for training 6.2.2 Prioritize requests for training 6.2.4 Assess needs for training 6.2.5 Identify existing resources that meet training needs 6.2.6 Use learning theory to develop or adapt training programs 6.2.7 Develop training plan 6.2.8 Implement training sessions and programs 6.2.9 Use a variety of resources and strategies 6.2.10 Evaluate impact of training programs	

Competency	Entry	Advanced 1	Advanced 2
6.3 Serve as a health education consultant	6.3.1 Assess needs for assistance 6.3.2 Prioritize requests for assistance 6.3.3 Define parameters of effective consultative relationships 6.3.4 Establish consultative relationships 6.3.6 Facilitate collaborative efforts to achieve program goals 6.3.8 Apply ethical principles in consultative relationships	6.3.5 Provide expert assistance 6.3.7 Evaluate the effectiveness of the expert assistance provided	

Area VII: Communicate and Advocate for Health and Health Education

The role.

Health education specialists are charged with the responsibility of providing information to diverse audiences. Whether through individual, small group, or mass communication techniques, health education specialists use their professional background to interpret and prioritize needs for health information and advocacy efforts (see Table 3.8). They also communicate to others the unique foundations of, and contributions offered by, health education professionals across a range of employment settings. To that end, health education specialists consider the value systems of the intended audience in delivering messages using a variety of strategies, methods and techniques, as well as engaging in health education advocacy. Through advocacy and promoting the profession, health education specialists promote health for individuals, groups, and communities.

Settings.

The following text describes how communication and advocacy are used in different health education practice settings.

Community setting. In a community setting, for example, lay health education specialists (also referred to as promotores, community health advocates, and community health advisors) might act as lay health education specialists for an asthma program reducing environmental triggers in the home. The health education specialist would work with the lay health education specialists to develop asset maps of the community, define goals and objectives, and develop program materials in appropriate languages at appropriate reading levels. The health education specialist would recruit, train and support the lay health workers as they conduct health education-related activities. Health education specialists can also act as advocates for community health needs, such as lobbying the local government to use funds in ways that help promote the community's health, or to create local laws or ordinances that promote community health.

School (K-12) setting. When employed in a school setting, a health education specialist might be responsible for promoting the coordinated school health approach by presenting curriculum information and student health information needs and concerns to groups of parents. In the event of parental concerns, the health education specialist would take into consideration the multiple value systems represented by the group and would employ appropriate strategies to communicate the material and respond to parents' questions. Depending on the topic, the health education specialist might use illustrations from classroom instruction, student presentations, videos, or Web technology to enhance the presentation. Health education specialists can also advocate for student or faculty health in a school setting by creating school health councils, or by suggesting ways to modify a curriculum.

Health care setting. In this setting, the health education specialist might be responsible for a program to support patients' smoking cessation efforts. The health education specialist would need to communicate with providers the importance of the program, as well as the health education specialist's appropriateness for launching such an effort. The health education specialist could advocate for corporate responsibility to engage in health promotion and prevention efforts. With the providers' understanding and support, the health education specialist would be responsible for informing the priority population of the program's availability in ways consistent with organizational policy and the values of the intended audience. Brochures, posters, flyers, public service announcements, and various electronic media might be considered.

Business/industry setting. A health education specialist employed in the workplace might become aware of some previously unrecognized health need among workers. The health education specialist would communicate that need (e.g., insufficient opportunity for physical activity) to management. Using his or her background in behavioral and biological sciences, the health education specialist would interpret the problem for management and articulate the possible ways of addressing the problem, such as offering a program or screening, or changing organizational policy. Acknowledging concerns specific to management, the health education specialist could then communicate ways in which a health education program or policy might benefit management and the worker.

College/university setting. A health education specialist in a college/university setting might be faced with the challenge of ensuring health education's "place" in the college curriculum. Recognizing multiple perspectives on expected student learning outcomes, the health education specialist would consider colleagues' professional backgrounds and use that information in formulating presentations on the importance of health education programs in the university environment. Communication might be handled through reports to curriculum committees, presentations to administrators, electronic communications or small group discussions with students and faculty. University health education specialists may develop an advocacy plan in order to improve the health of current and future students.

University health services setting. In a university health services setting, the health education specialist interfaces with students, health care providers, faculty, and other stakeholders. In this arena, the health education specialist might be charged with providing an educational program or social norm campaign to improve students' decision-making about use of drugs and alcohol. The health education specialist would communicate to health care providers the need for such a campaign, and contribute to the program to ensure the providers' support and participation. The health education specialist would communicate the educational purpose of the program and/or relevant social norms data to students and interpret its value relative to their health education needs and concerns. This communication could be handled through electronic or print channels to individual students, posters placed around campus, and presentations before small groups within dormitories. The health education specialist might also work with select student organizations to encourage policy development regarding alcohol consumption on campus, alternatives to alcohol consumption, and advocate for local laws or ordinances that stiffen alcohol or drug-related offenses for businesses.

Table 3.8

Health Educator Job Analysis 2010 Model: Area VII: Communicate and advocate for health and health education

Competency	Entry	Advanced 1	Advanced 2
7.1 Assess and prioritize health information and advocacy needs	7.1.1 Identify current and emerging issues that may influence health and health education 7.1.2 Access accurate resources related to identified issues 7.1.3 Analyze the impact of existing and proposed policies on health 7.1.4 Analyze factors that influence decision-makers		
7.2 Identify and develop a variety of communication strategies, methods, and techniques	7.2.1 Create messages using communication theories and models 7.2.2 Tailor messages to priority populations 7.2.3 Incorporate images to enhance messages 7.2.4 Select effective methods or channels for communicating to priority populations 7.2.5 Pilot test messages and delivery methods with priority populations 7.2.6 Revise messages based on pilot feedback		

Competency	Entry	Advanced 1	Advanced 2
7.3 Deliver messages using a variety of strategies, methods and techniques	7.3.1 Use techniques that empower individuals and communities to improve their health 7.3.2 Employ technology to communicate to priority populations 7.3.3 Evaluate the delivery of communication strategies, methods, and techniques		
7.4 Engage in health education advocacy	7.4.1 Engage stakeholders in advocacy 7.4.2 Develop an advocacy plan in compliance with local, state, and/or federal policies and procedures 7.4.3 Comply with organizational policies related to participating in advocacy 7.4.4 Communicate the impact of health and health education on organizational and socio-ecological factors 7.4.5 Use data to support advocacy messages 7.4.6 Implement advocacy plans 7.4.7 Incorporate media and technology in advocacy 7.4.8 Participate in advocacy initiatives		7.4.9 Lead advocacy initiatives 7.4.10 Evaluate advocacy efforts
7.5 Influence policy to promote health	7.5.2 Identify the significance and implications of health policy for individuals, groups, and communities 7.5.3 Advocate for health-related policies, regulations, laws, or rules 7.5.5 Employ policy and media advocacy techniques to influence decision-makers		7.5.1 Use evaluation and research findings in policy analysis 7.5.4 Use evidence-based research to develop policies to promote health

Competency	Entry	Advanced 1	Advanced 2
7.6 Promote the health education profession	7.6.1 Develop a personal plan for professional growth and service 7.6.2 Describe state-of-the-art health education practice 7.6.3 Explain the major responsibilities of the health education specialist in the practice of health education 7.6.4 Explain the role of health education associations in advancing the profession 7.6.5 Explain the benefits of participating in professional organizations 7.6.6 Facilitate professional growth of self and others 7.6.7 Explain the history of the health education profession and its current and future implications for professional practice 7.6.8 Explain the role of credentialing in the promotion of the health education profession 7.6.9 Engage in professional development activities 7.6.10 Serve as a mentor to others 7.6.11 Develop materials that contribute to the professional literature 7.6.12 Engage in service to advance the health education profession		

Section IV:
Using the HEJA 2010 Model

Section IV: Using the HEJA 2010 Model

The CUP Model (NCHEC, SOPHE, & AAHE, 2006), the predecessor to the HEJA 2010 Model, was used to establish common standards of practice in a hierarchical framework for health education specialists. The model has been used by a variety of stakeholders to more clearly define, develop, and apply the Competencies and Sub-competencies of the profession. The HEJA 2010 Model will serve the profession in a similar manner, but will likely do so in more precise terms due to the expanded list of Sub-competencies and refined advanced-level components that were validated in the HEJA 2010 study. Potential applications and benefits of the HEJA 2010 Model for selected stakeholder groups are described below, followed by a set of formal recommendations to the profession that were endorsed by the boards of the Society for Public Health Education (SOPHE), the American Association for Health Education (AAHE), the National Commission for Health Education Credentialing (NCHEC), the National Implementation Task Force for Accreditation in Health Education, and the Coalition of National Health Education Organizations.

Health education students

Choosing a career path can be a daunting and confusing process. This is particularly true for the individual entering a university system for the first time, with limited experience in work settings associated with the wide variety of available career options. The HEJA 2010 Model, like its predecessor, can be useful to prospective students who are interested in a career in health education. The model can be used to develop a basic understanding of the Competencies and Sub-competencies commonly used by health education specialists, and can serve as a guide for exploring the various work settings in which they can be applied. Students who are considering a graduate degree in the field will be better prepared to make the decision and choose a program if they are familiar with the entry- and advanced-level distinctions in the model. The model can also be compared to the stated Competencies of other professions to help understand professional distinctions.

Students enrolled in health education degree programs can use the model as a guide for self-directed learning and assessment. It can be used to set personal achievement goals specific to each Area of Responsibility and assess progress toward mastering each Area. The student can use model Competencies and Sub-competencies as a guide for selecting and evaluating degree programs and specific courses; and can actively seek opportunities to serve as a volunteer, intern, and/or employee in activities and settings that will help gain actual experience in a specific Area of Responsibility. The model can be used as a framework in preparing for the national examination to become a Certified Health Education Specialist (CHES) or Master Certified Health Education Specialist (MCHES). The framework can also be used to create a professional portfolio and resumé that reflect experiences and demonstrated abilities relevant to the profession.

College and university faculty members

Like its predecessor, the HEJA 2010 Model can be used by faculty of university degree programs in curriculum development, student mentoring, and program accreditation efforts. A competency-based approach to curriculum development can enhance the marketability of program graduates and is an established standard for achieving formal approval/accreditation for health education programs. Faculty members and their students can benefit when expectations for student performance, and faculty teaching and mentoring, are clearly defined within the model framework. The model can be used to develop program goals and objectives; course descriptions, syllabi, and evaluation instruments; student handbooks and specific guides for practica/internships and portfolios; and assessment tools for program approval and accreditation. The model can also be useful when comparing the stated competencies of other professional degrees offered by a university, and in developing program descriptions and marketing materials. Furthermore, it can be used to communicate program needs to university administrators and leverage resources and opportunities for program development. Faculty members are encouraged to seek and maintain approval/accreditation relevant to their degree programs and to conduct periodic reviews to assess and maintain relevance and currency in their programs (see Appendix D for matrices for analyzing curricula).

Health education practitioners

Practicing health education specialists can use the HEJA 2010 Model as a guide for professional development. Continuing education is not only a requirement for CHES and MCHES, but it is also essential for the practicing health education specialist to remain current, effective, and marketable in the field. The HEJA 2010 Model (and future versions of the model) can be used to help the practitioner monitor changes in Competencies and Sub-competencies as they emerge, self-assess areas of needed renewal and new skill development, and select professional development opportunities directed toward current practices in the profession. Practitioners who are interested in changing work settings and/or in promoting to more advanced-levels of practice will be better equipped to do so if they are aware of and skilled in the generic entry-level and relevant advanced-level Competencies represented in the model.

Professional development providers

Leaders of organizations and agencies that provide continuing education and professional development opportunities will benefit from using the HEJA 2010 Model as a guide. Health education practitioners often look to these organizations and agencies as a source for staying current in an evolving professional field. As the number of CHES continues to grow, and as the newly-developed master-level certification (MCHES) is initiated, the demand for competency-based professional development opportunities is expected to increase. Opportunities to renew and develop new skills represented in the HEJA 2010 Model will be critical to the future of a growing and evolving health education profession.

Other health professionals

The previously established CUP Model has contributed to a growing understanding and appreciation for health education specialists among members of other health professions. The HEJA 2010 Model can be used to further promote the growing appreciation for health education specialists and their valuable roles in health-related partnerships.

Health education employers

Most Competencies of health education specialists are adaptable to a variety of work-related projects. Some Competencies enable a health education specialist to be the "glue" that bonds other health specialists and communities together as well as the facilitator of goal achievement in health-promoting partnerships. The HEJA 2010 Model, which contains an updated, empirically validated description of current practice at all three levels, will be useful in furthering an appreciation for and employment of health education specialists. Employers should be encouraged to use the HEJA 2010 Model when developing position announcements and job descriptions, supporting and requiring professional development for their employed health education specialists, and evaluating employee performance. Because the CHES and MCHES credentials reflect mastery of current entry- and advanced-level Responsibilities and Competencies, employers are also encouraged to employ individuals with these certifications.

Leaders of professional credentialing and program accreditation

The HEJA 2010 Model should serve as the standard for individual credentialing and program approval or accreditation. Because the HEJA 2010 Model contains more Sub-competencies and some additional Competencies than the CUP Model, it will require the development of specific items for the current CHES and pending MCHES exams, and adjustments to criteria for program approval and accreditation. These changes should enhance the profession's ability to assess and promote individual Competencies and program quality based on a more precise and expanded definition of Competencies and Sub-competencies. Inclusion of the entry-level (generic) Competencies at all levels of credentialing and accreditation, and the addition of the advanced-level Competencies in criteria used for advanced-level credentialing and professional preparation, will be important.

Policy makers and funding agencies

The HEJA 2010 Model can be used by policy makers in governmental and non-governmental settings to establish organizational policies related to health education efforts. These policies can impact the development of health programs and interventions and the criteria for funding projects and research. The model's expanded version of Competencies and Sub-competencies further clarifies the distinctive role of health education specialists at entry- and advanced-levels of practice. It should be used by the U.S. Department of Labor and the states implementing the Standard Occupational Classification system to collect data and monitor the evolving nature and job outlook for health education specialists.

Recommendations to the Profession

The HEJA 2010 outcomes have significant implications for professional certification, preparation, continuing education, and practice in the health education profession. In 2009, the boards of SOPHE, AAHE, and NCHEC issued six recommendations for using the HEJA 2010 Model. These recommendations also were endorsed by the CNHEO and the National Implementation Task Force for Accreditation in Health Education in 2010. The recommendations build on earlier studies and reports for the field, which revealed a lack of clarity and unity on central tenets related to health education quality assurance and credentialing, and the acknowledgement of the following key principles: a) Health education is a single profession, with common roles and responsibilities; b) Professional preparation in health education provides the health education specialist with knowledge and skills that form a foundation of common and setting-specific Competencies; c) Accreditation is the primary quality assurance mechanism in higher education; and d) The health education profession is responsible for assuring quality in professional preparation and practice. Thus, to continue to advance the field, the following recommendations should provide a basis and direction for all future efforts:

1. Baccalaureate programs in health education should prepare health education graduates to perform all seven of the health education Responsibilities, 34 Competencies and 162 Sub-competencies identified as entry-level in the HEJA 2010 hierarchical model.
2. NCHEC should use all seven health education Responsibilities, 34 Competencies and 162 Sub-competencies identified as entry-level in the 2010 hierarchical model as the basis for revisions to the entry-level CHES (CHES) examination.
3. Graduate programs in health education should ensure the preparation of health education graduates to perform all seven of the health education Responsibilities, 34 Competencies and 223 Sub-competencies (162 entry-level and 61 advanced-level) in the HEJA 2010 hierarchical model.
4. NCHEC should use the advanced-level Responsibilities, Competencies and Sub-competencies for the new advanced-level exam (MCHES).
5. All of the Responsibilities, Competencies and Sub-competences should be used for professional development activities.
6. Accrediting and approval bodies should be encouraged to recognize the 2010 HEJA Responsibilities, Competencies and Sub-competencies as the basis for quality assurance for professional preparation programs.

Profession-wide support of these six recommendations can significantly impact the future of the health education profession. For example, the HEJA 2010 Model is already in use by NCHEC leaders to develop specifications for the pending MCHES examination. The HEJA 2010 Model can also be useful in current efforts to develop a unified or coordinated approach to accreditation for professional preparation programs. Professional development and continuing education can be expanded to include appropriate levels of learning for those in advanced-levels of practice. As with the CUP Model, the HEJA 2010 Model and methods used in the analysis can serve as a guide upon which future Competency updates can be designed. The regular, periodic re-verification of the health education Responsibilities, Competencies, and Sub-competencies is a process that is iterative and necessary to ensure that certification, preparation and professional development are based on what is needed in current practice. It is recommended that this re-verification process be completed every five years.

Section V:
Changes in the Responsibilities, Competencies, and Sub-competencies of Health Education Specialists from 1985 to 2010

Section V: Changes in the Responsibilities, Competencies, and Sub-competencies of Health Education Specialists from 1985 to 2010

This 2010 publication marks the 25th year since the role of entry-level health education specialists and their related scope of practice were first established within Seven Areas of Responsibility. Though the HEJA 2010 Model marks the second time in which changes were made to that original framework to adapt to emerging changes in current practice, the original Seven Areas of Responsibility have largely remained intact. Table 5.1 illustrates how the profession began with seven areas in 1985, added three graduate-level areas (Areas VIII-X) in 1999, and combined the original seven from 1985 and three graduate-level areas from 1999 into an updated seven areas in 2006. The refined Seven Areas of Responsibility in the HEJA 2010 Model are also provided in the table. As stated by the CUP Model authors, this constant in health education practice "…is a testament to the solid foundations on which the profession stands" (NCHEC, SOPHE, & AAHE, 2006, p. 48).

The three-tiered hierarchical framework of entry- and advanced-level practice that emerged in the CUP Model was also validated through the HEJA 2010 study, along with a large number of Competencies and Sub-competencies that were part of the original CUP Model. However, as was true regarding CUP study outcomes, outcomes of the HEJA 2010 study revealed the need for wording changes to some model components, the reassignment of some Competencies and Sub-competencies, and the addition of new Competencies and Sub-competencies to more accurately reflect the evolving practice of entry- and advanced-level health education specialists. The new numbering system (see Section III) is an additional change that can be noted in the model and in descriptions below. These descriptions include a brief overview of changes made in the HEJA 2010 Model compared to the CUP Model. A more detailed analysis of changes is represented in the grid provided in Appendix B entitled Comparison of the Areas of Responsibility, Competencies, and Sub-competencies of the CUP Model and the HEJA 2010 Model

Seven Areas of Responsibility

Outcomes of the HEJA 2010 study validated the continued use of the seven areas established in the CUP Model with some minor revisions made to the wording of the Areas of Responsibility. Despite minor changes in wording, the first four Areas of Responsibility have retained their primary foci: *Assess, Plan, Implement, and Evaluate.* The HEJA 2010 Task Force used the analysis opportunity to empirically determine whether "research" and "evaluation" components of Area IV should be separated. Study results concluded that the two should remain within the same area with some research-specific Sub-competencies designated as "advanced-level." In Area V, the words *and Manage* were added to the original word *Administer* to more closely reflect some subtle distinctions between the two concepts. The wording for Areas VI and VII were retained from the CUP Model. Changes specific to each Area and the advanced- levels are described below.

Table 5.1

Comparison of Areas of Responsibility (1985 – 2010)

Entry-Level Framework (1985)	Graduate-Level Framework (1999)	CUP Model (2006)	HEJA Model (2010)
I. Assessing individual and community needs for health education	I. Assessing individual and community needs for health education	I. Assess individual and community needs for health education	I. Assess needs, assets, and capacity for health education
II. Planning effective health education programs	II. Planning effective health education programs	II. Plan health education strategies, interventions, and programs	II. Plan health education
III. Implementing health education programs	III. Implementing health education programs	III. Implement health education strategies, interventions, and programs	III. Implement health education
IV. Evaluating effectiveness of health education programs	IV. Evaluating effectiveness of health education programs	IV. Conduct evaluation and research related to health education	IV. Conduct evaluation and research related to health education
V. Coordinating provision of health education services	V. Coordinating provision of health education services	V. Administer health education strategies, interventions, and programs	V. Administer and manage health education
VI. Acting as a resource person in health education	VI. Acting as a resource person in health education	VI. Serve as a health education resource person	VI. Serve as a health education resource person
VII. Communicating health and health education needs, concerns, and resources	VII. Communicating health and health education needs, concerns, and resources	VII. Communicate and advocate for health and health education	VII. Communicate and advocate for health and health education
	VIII. Applying appropriate research principles and techniques in health education		
	IX. Administering health education programs		
	X. Advancing the profession of health education		

Note. Adapted from *Overview of the National Health Educator Competencies Updated Project, 1998-2004* by Gilmore, Olsen, Taub, and Connell (2005).

SECTION: V.

Area of Responsibility I: Assess needs, assets, and capacity for health education.

Under Area of Responsibility I, a new Competency 1.1, *Plan assessment process*, emerged from the HEJA 2010 study. The majority of the remaining Competencies and Sub-competencies from the CUP Model were retained but "shifted" to the next consecutive letter in the Competency sequence. For example, the former *Competency A: Access existing health-related data* from the CUP Model was slightly re-worded and is now *Competency 1.2: Access existing information and data related to health* in the HEJA 2010 Model. The original *Competency B: Collect health-related data* was re-worded to emphasize inclusion of quantitative and qualitative data and became the following Competency in the HEJA 2010 Model: *Competency 1.3: Collect quantitative and/or qualitative data related to health*. The addition of a new Competency 1.1 and the shifting of original Competencies resulted in a net increase of one Competency in Area I.

Area of Responsibility II: Plan health education.

Though the label of Area of Responsibility II was significantly simplified (from *Plan Health Education Strategies, Interventions, and Programs* in the CUP Model to *Plan Health Education* in the HEJA 2010 Model), only minor changes were needed in the Competencies and Sub-competencies to adapt to HEJA 2010 study outcomes. For example, the wording of the original Competency A (now Competency 1.2) was changed from "*Involve people and organizations*" to "*Involve priority populations and other stakeholders*" *in the planning process*. Elements of the original Competency B concept of incorporating principles of community organization were incorporated into Competency 2.1 within that same Area and into some elements of assessment (Area I), and implementation (Area III). Other Competencies were shifted in sequence to match a common flow of tasks (e.g., involve priority populations, develop goals and objectives, select or design strategies, develop a scope and sequence of delivery).

Area of Responsibility III: Implement health education.

Some major changes to the integration of *ethical practice* into the HEJA 2010 Model significantly impacted Area of Responsibility III. In the CUP Model, the original *Competency C: Use a variety of methods to implement strategies, interventions, and programs* included a single Sub-competency that focused on ethical practice: *Use the Code of Ethics in professional practice*. The HEJA 2010 study outcomes validated that ethical practice is an important Sub-competency within the context of a variety of Competencies in the model. Thus, this Competency was replaced with the addition of eight ethics-related Sub-competencies integrated into various Areas of Responsibility throughout the model.

Area of Responsibility IV: Conduct evaluation and research related to health education.

In Area of Responsibility IV, the original *Competency E: Interpret Results from Evaluation and Research*, was shifted to become *Competency 4.4: Interpret results of the evaluation/research* in the HEJA 2010 Model. Elements of the original *Competency F: Infer implications from findings for future health-related activities*, which had Sub-competencies at the advanced 1- and 2-levels only in the CUP Model, were integrated into Competency (4.4.) of the HEJA 2010 Model. The older, separate, Competency F of the CUP Model was replaced with a new *Competency 4.5: Apply findings from evaluation/research.*

Area of Responsibility V: Administer and manage health education.

The HEJA 2010 study outcomes indicated that some Competencies and Sub-competencies may be more commonly labeled as "management" rather than "administration" in some work settings. A number of existing and new Sub-competencies were validated at entry and advanced levels in Area of Responsibility V. For instance, a new Competency was added to this area: *Competency 5.5: Facilitate partnerships in support of health education.* Though only one Sub-competency, *Facilitate partner relationship(s)* was validated for Competency 5.5 at the entry level, four advanced-level Sub-competencies were validated including: *identify potential partner(s), assess capacity of potential partner(s) to meet program goals, elicit feedback from partner(s), and evaluate feasibility of continuing partnership.*

Area of Responsibility VI: Serve as a health education resource person.

Area of Responsibility VI was expanded to include a substantial number of new advanced-level Sub-competencies that focus on training and serving as a consultant. A new *Competency 6.2: Provide training* with one entry-level and nine advanced-level Sub-competencies was validated for HEJA 2010 model inclusion. The original *Competency D: Establish consultative relationships* in the CUP Model was re-worded as Competency 6.3: *Serve as a health education consultant* and expanded to include more Sub-competencies.

Area of Responsibility VII: Communicate and advocate for health and health education.

Area of Responsibility VII in the HEJA 2010 Model contains two more Competencies than the CUP Model and significant wording changes Of particular importance are additional Sub-competencies in *Competency 7.4: Influence policy to promote health* (formerly *Competency D* in the CUP Model), and *Competency 7.6: Promote the health education profession* (formerly *Competency F*).

Advanced-level Competencies and Sub-Competencies

The three distinct levels of practice established through the CUP study were verified in the HEJA 2010 study. These three levels were identified as entry (less than five years of experience and a baccalaureate or master degree), advanced 1 (five or more years of experience and a baccalaureate or master degree), and advanced 2 (five or more years of experience and a doctoral degree). Consistent with CUP findings, these practice levels are hierarchical in the HEJA 2010 Model. The Sub-competencies in the advanced 1-level include those in the entry-level (generic Sub-competencies) plus additional Sub-competencies specific to advanced 1-level practice. The Sub-competencies in the advanced 2-level include *generic* (entry-level) Sub-competencies, advanced 1-level Sub-competencies, and an additional set of Sub-competencies specific to advanced 2-level practice.

The levels of practice at which some Sub-competencies were validated for the HEJA 2010 Model differed from level-specific assignments in the CUP Model. The CUP Model contained 163 Sub-competencies that constituted 82 entry-level, 48 advanced 1-level, and

33 advanced 2-level Sub-competencies. Of the 223 Sub-competencies validated for the HEJA 2010 Model, 162 were generic or entry-level, 42 were advanced 1-level, and 19 were advanced 2-level. As previously explained, the number of Sub-competencies was expanded to include more Sub-competencies related to applied ethics, training, serving as a consultant, and facilitating partnerships.

Though the number and general nature of advanced 1-level Sub-competencies remained largely the same when comparing the CUP Model to the HEJA 2010 Model, fewer Sub-competencies in the HEJA 2010 Model were validated as being unique to the advanced 2-level than were included at only that level in the CUP Model. For example, the CUP Model included advanced 2-level Sub-competencies related to assessment (e.g., critique sources of health information, assess the learning environment), planning (e.g., formulate a variety of education methods, match proposed learning activities with stated program objectives, select appropriate theory-based strategies in health program planning), implementation (e.g., use a variety of educational methods, use instructional resources that meet a variety of training needs), and serving as a resource (e.g., describe consulting skills needed by health education specialists) that were integrated into and validated as generic or entry-level Sub-competencies in the HEJA 2010 Model.

In addition, some Sub-competencies deemed exclusive to the advanced 2-level in the CUP Model were validated as advanced 1-level Sub-competencies for the HEJA 2010 Model. For example, some administration-related Sub-competencies (e.g., facilitate administration of the evaluation plan, prepare proposals to obtain fiscal resources) were integrated into and validated as advanced 1-level Sub-competencies.

It is important to note that the inclusion of these Sub-competencies in the entry-and advanced 1-levels of the HEJA 2010 Model is only an indicator that the practice of these Sub-competencies is not exclusive to advanced 2-level of practice. By definition, health education specialists at the advanced 2-level practice all Sub-competencies in the HEJA 2010 Model, including those in the entry- and advanced 1-levels, along with the 19 validated in the HEJA 2010 study as being exclusively practiced at the advanced 2-level.

When comparing the Sub-competencies across the three levels within the HEJA 2010 Model, it is notable that Sub-competencies practiced exclusively at the advanced 2-level were mostly those related to research, the professional dissemination of research findings, and using research and evaluation outcomes to influence policy. Advanced 1-level Sub-competencies, that were practiced by advanced 1-and advanced 2-level health education specialists but not entry-level specialists were predominantly related to administrative and management roles. ◆

Section VI:
Core Knowledge Items

Section VI: Core Knowledge Items

The ability to effectively perform a professional competency is dependent, in part, on one's mastery of relevant knowledge; however, clearly defining knowledge bases that are essential and generic to a competency-based framework can be a challenge. For the first time in the history of the health education profession, a knowledge-based survey was integrated into the HEJA 2010 study to identify and validate core knowledge items for use in various aspects of professional preparation, credentialing, and professional development efforts.

As indicated in Section II, 115 knowledge items were generated through a modified Delphi technique in Phase 1 of the HEJA 2010 study. These items were included in the HEJA survey implemented in Phase 2. A 4-point rating scale based on the Revised Bloom's Taxonomy (Anderson & Krathwohl, 2001) was used by health education specialists who rated these items in terms of cognitive levels of use in their work (*I do not use the knowledge, I recognize and/or recall the knowledge, I apply and/or integrate the knowledge, I use the knowledge to evaluate and/or create*). One hundred thirteen of the items were used by at least 50% of participants and included in the knowledge item list provided on the following pages.

A volunteer team of health education specialists with expertise in competency development and credentialing reviewed each knowledge item and assigned it to at least one of the Seven Areas of Responsibility in the HEJA 2010 Model. The 113 knowledge items are listed in alphabetical order in Table 6.1. The asterisk for each knowledge item designates the Area(s) of Responsibility to which it was linked by the specialists. This table can be used by university faculty who teach courses to which one or more of the Seven Areas of Responsibility have been assigned. The course instructor should ensure that the designated knowledge items for that Area of Responsibility are addressed in the assigned course (or in course prerequisites) so that students will be equipped with knowledge needed to address related Competencies. Leaders of professional development efforts can use the table in the same manner so that knowledge bases linked to specific Areas of Responsibility are incorporated into professional development events. Students and individual practitioners can also use the table as a guide for understanding and addressing needed knowledge bases when preparing for certification examinations or in self-guided professional development efforts.

The 113 validated knowledge items are not considered an exhaustive representation of all essential core knowledge, and some items on the list may overlap in some ways; however, each item on the list was empirically validated as essential to the work of at least 50% of health education specialists who participated in the study. As such, the list of core knowledge can serve as a useful first step in establishing core knowledge items that are essential to the competency-based framework for health education specialists. Additional research in future job analyses is recommended to further explore and develop a broad knowledge base that is generic and essential to the practice of health education specialists.

Table 6.1

Validated knowledge items by Area of Responsibility

	VALIDATED KNOWLEDGE ITEM	Area I	Area II	Area III	Area IV	Area V	Area VI	Area VII
001	Advocacy strategies		*					*
002	Advocacy techniques		*					*
003	Basic elements of US health care, public health and education systems	*	*					*
004	Behavior change concepts [005, 040]**	*	*	*			*	
005	Behavior change strategies [004, 040]**	*	*	*			*	
006	Biopsychosocial models of health and disease	*	*				*	
007	Capacity building techniques	*	*	*		*	*	*
008	Characteristics of data (reliability, validity, fairness, unbiased)	*			*			
009	Characteristics of different organizations/agencies (e.g., governmental, quasi-governmental, voluntary, professional)		*	*			*	
010	Coaching techniques					*		
011	Coalition building [018, 019, 080]**		*	*		*	*	*
012	Collaboration strategies	*	*	*		*	*	
013	Collaborative health services	*	*	*		*	*	
014	Communication channels		*	*				*
015	Communication styles	*	*	*	*	*	*	*
016	Communication techniques	*		*	*	*	*	*
017	Communication theory	*	*				*	*
018	Community building [011, 019, 080]**		*	*			*	*
019	Community organization [011, 018, 080]**		*	*			*	*
020	Conflict resolution techniques		*	*		*		
021	Consulting principles						*	
022	Cost-analyses (cost-identification, cost-benefit, cost-effectiveness, and cost utility analysis)		*		*			
023	Credentialing in health education							*
024	Data collection instruments and methods	*			*			
025	Databases (literature and data) [059]**	*			*		*	

	VALIDATED KNOWLEDGE ITEM	Area I	Area II	Area III	Area IV	Area V	Area VI	Area VII
026	Descriptive statistics	*			*			
027	Education theory		*	*				
028	Educational resources (e.g., audiovisual equipment, computers, curriculum) and criteria for selection (e.g., age and culture appropriateness, readability, learning style)		*	*			*	
029	Elements of a health education program (e.g., framework, scope and sequence goals, objectives, time line, budget, evaluation, resources)	*	*	*	*	*		*
030	Epidemiological principles and methods	*			*		*	
031	Ethical principles and behavior	*	*	*	*	*	*	*
032	Evaluation models		*		*			
033	Factors influencing health (e.g., medical care, genetics, behavioral, social, environmental)	*	*				*	*
034	Financial management (e.g., budgeting, revenue forecasting)					*		
035	Fund raising methods and techniques					*		
036	Global health issues						*	*
037	Grant proposal writing	*	*	*	*	*		*
038	Group dynamics	*	*	*	*	*	*	*
039	Group facilitation techniques	*	*	*	*	*	*	*
040	Health behavior theory [004, 005]**	*	*	*		*		
041	Health disparities	*	*				*	*
042	Health education professional associations							*
043	Health impact assessments	*			*			
044	Health literacy [058]**	*	*	*	*		*	*
045	Health numeracy	*	*	*	*		*	*
046	Health risk appraisals (health assessments)	*			*			
047	Human resources (e.g., hiring, supervision, evaluation, dismissal)				*	*		
048	Inequities leading to disparities	*	*				*	*
049	Inferential statistics	*			*			
050	Informatics	*	*		*	*		
051	Institutional Review Boards and human subjects review committees	*			*			
052	Laws, rules, and regulations related to health education practice	*	*	*	*	*	*	*

VALIDATED KNOWLEDGE ITEM	Area I	Area II	Area III	Area IV	Area V	Area VI	Area VII
053 Leadership concepts and theories					*		
054 Legal issues impacting health education (e.g., privacy, Health Insurance Portability and Accountability (HIPAA) informed consent, and disability laws)	*	*	*	*	*	*	*
055 Legislative process and political structures	*	*	*	*	*	*	*
056 Legislative theory/policy development and processes	*	*				*	*
057 Levels of measurement	*			*			
058 Linguistic characteristics of population groups and demographic groups [044]**							*
059 Literature search techniques [025]**	*			*		*	
060 Logic models	*	*	*	*			
061 Management theory and strategies					*		
062 Marketing principles and techniques		*	*				*
063 Marketing theory	*	*	*				
064 Mentoring techniques					*		*
065 Methods for distributing educational materials		*	*			*	
066 Methods of reporting data (e.g., graphs, charts, tables, narrative)	*	*		*			
067 Multiple dimensions of health	*	*				*	
068 Needs assessment techniques	*						
069 Organizational change theory		*	*		*	*	
070 Organizations and agencies that provide various types of health information, health services and expertise		*	*			*	
071 Participatory research techniques	*			*			
072 Pedagogy [073]**		*	*				
073 Pedagogical concepts [072]**	*	*	*			*	
074 Performance-based assessment					*		
075 Pilot testing techniques	*	*	*	*			*
076 Planning models	*	*					
077 Policy development processes		*					*
078 Practice-based evidence [082]**	*	*	*	*	*	*	*
079 Primary, secondary, and tertiary levels of prevention	*	*				*	

	VALIDATED KNOWLEDGE ITEM	Area I	Area II	Area III	Area IV	Area V	Area VI	Area VII
080	Principles of community organizing and building [011, 018, 019]**	*	*			*		
081	Principles of cultural competence	*	*	*	*	*	*	*
082	Principles of evidence-based practice [078]**	*	*	*	*	*	*	*
083	Professional code of ethics	*	*	*	*	*	*	*
084	Professional development opportunities							*
085	Professional literature, including current research, trends, issues	*	*	*	*	*	*	*
086	Professional terminology	*	*	*	*	*	*	*
087	Program evaluation techniques	*	*		*			
088	Program implementation processes and methods			*	*			
089	Program management techniques and principles (e.g., supervision, staying within budget)			*				
090	Programming planning techniques		*				*	
091	Public relations					*	*	*
092	Qualitative data analysis techniques	*			*			
093	Quantitative data analysis techniques	*			*			
094	Relation among theory, research and practice	*	*	*	*			
095	Research design and methods				*			
096	Roles of health and related professionals						*	*
097	Roles of the health educator						*	*
098	Sampling plans and techniques	*			*			
099	Social justice	*	*	*	*	*	*	*
100	Sources of social, physical, political, cultural, and economic information	*	*	*	*	*	*	*
101	Standards for education	*	*	*	*	*	*	*
102	Statistical techniques and terms	*			*			
103	Strategic planning process					*		
104	Strategies for identifying and involving community organizations, resources, and participants	*	*		*	*	*	*
105	Strengths, Weaknesses, Opportunities, Threats (SWOT) analysis	*	*		*	*		
106	Systems theory	*	*	*		*		

SECTION: VI

#	Item	I	II	III	IV	V	VI	VII
107	Team building	*	*	*	*	*	*	*
108	Training methods and techniques	*	*	*	*	*	*	
109	Types of data (e.g., primary and secondary, qualitative and quantitative)	*			*		*	
110	Types of evaluation (e.g., formative, process, outcome, summative, impact)	*	*		*			
111	Types of timetables for planning		*	*			*	
112	Use of technology in practice	*	*	*	*		*	*
113	Volunteer recruitment and management techniques					*		

Note. Area I-Assess needs, assets, and capacity for health education; Area II-Plan health education; Area III-Implement health education; Area IV-Conduct evaluation and research related to health education; Area V-Administer and manage health education; Area VI-Serve as a health education resource person; Area VII-Communicate and advocate for health and health education. Knowledge item(s) link(s) to specific Area(s) of Responsibility are indicated by an asterisk (*)

Knowledge item in brackets [ ] and marked with** indicates that the items are closely related.

SECTION: VI

References:

Airhihenbuwa, C. O., Cottrell, R. R., Adeyanju, M., Auld, M. E., Lysoby, L., & Smith, B. J. (2005). The National Health Educator Competencies Update Project: Celebrating a milestone and recommending next steps to the profession. *Health Education & Behavior, 32*, 722-724.

Ali, A. K. (2005). Using the Delphi technique to search for empirical measures for local planning agency power. *The Qualitative Report, 10*(4), 717-744.

Allegrante, J. P., Airhihenbuwa, C. O., Auld, M. E., Birch, D. B., Roe, K. M., Smith, B. J. (2004). Toward a unified system of accreditation for professional preparation in health education: Final report of the National Task Force on Accreditation in Health Education. *Health Education and Behavior, 31*(6), 1-16.

Allegrante, J. P., Barry, M. M., Airhihenbuwa, C. O., Auld, M. E., Collins, J. L., Lamarre, M. C. et al. (2009). Domains of core competency, standards, and quality assurance for building global capacity in health promotion: The Galway Consensus conference statement. *Health Education & Behavior, 36*(3), 476-482.

American Association for Health Education, National Commission for Health Education Credentialing, & Society for Public Health Education. (1999). A competency-based framework for graduate-level health educators. Allentown, PA: Author.

Anderson, L., & Krathwohl, P., Eds. (2001) A taxonomy for learning, teaching, and assessing — A revision of Bloom's taxonomy of educational objectives. New York: Longman.

Battel-Kirk, B., Barry, M. M., Taub, A., and Lysoby, L. (2009). A review of the international literature on health promotion competencies: Identifying frameworks and core competencies. *Global Health Promotion, 16*(2), 12-20.

Benarie, M. (1988). Delphi and Delphi like approaches with special regard to environmental standard setting. *Technological Forecasting and Social Change, 40*(2), 149-158.

Bureau of Labor Statistics. (2007). *Occupational outlook handbook, 2008-09 edition.* Retrieved from: http://www.bls.gov/oco/ocos063.htm

Cottrell, R. R., Lysoby, L., Rasar King, L., Airhihenbuwa, C. O., Roe, K. M., and Allegrante, J. P. (2009). Current developments in accreditation and certification for health promotion and health education: A perspective on systems of quality assurance in the United States. *Health Education & Behavior, 36*(3), 451-463.

Council on Education for Public Health. (2005). *Accreditation criteria for public health programs.* Retrieved from http://www.ceph.org/files/public/PHP-Criteria-2005.SO5.pdf

Dennis, D. L., & Mahoney, B. S. (2008). The CHES examination: Standards and statistical information. *The CHES Bulletin*, 19(1), 11.

Gambescia, S. F., Cottrell, R. R., Capwell, E., Auld, M. E., Mullen, K., Lysoby, L., Goldsmith, M., & Smith, B. (2009). Marketing health educators to employers: Survey findings, interpretations, and considerations for the profession. *Health Promotion Practice*, 11(4), 495-504.

Gilmore, G. D., & Campbell, M. D. (2005). *Needs and capacity assessment strategies for health education and health promotion* (3rd ed.). Sudbury, MA: Jones & Bartlett.

Gilmore, G. D., Olsen, L.K., Taub, A., & Connell, D. (2005). Overview of the national health educator competencies update project 1998-2004. *Health Education & Behavior*, 32(6), 725-737.

Hambleton, R. J., & Rogers, H. K. (1986). Technical advances in credentialing examinations, *Evaluation and the Health Professions*, 9(2), 205-229.

Hezel Associates. (2007). *Marketing the health education profession: Knowledge, attitudes and hiring practices of employers*. Retrieved from: http://www.cnheo.org/PDF%20files/ExecSummary_Marketing%20the%20Health%20Education%20Profession%20%282%29.pdf

Howze, E. H., Auld, M. E., Woodhouse, L. D., Gershick, J., & Livingood, W. C. (2009). Building health promotion capacity in developing countries: Strategies from 60 years of experience in the United States. *Health Education & Behavior*, 36(3), 464-475.

Impara, J. C. (1995). *Licensure testing: Purposes, procedures, and practices*. Lincoln, NE: Buros Institute of Mental Measurement.

Institute for Credentialing Excellence. (2009). Standards. Retrieved from: http://www.credentialingexcellence.org/PublicationsandResources/Publications/Standards/tabid/390/Default.aspx

Joint Committee on Terminology. (2001). Report of the 2000 joint committee on health education and promotion terminology committee. *American Journal of Health Education*, 32(2), 89-103.

Livingood, W. C., & Auld, M. E. (2001). The credentialing of a population-based profession: Lessons learned from health education certification. *Journal of Public Health Management & Practice*, 7(4), 38-45.

National Commission for Certifying Agencies. (2005). *Application for certification program accreditation*. Washington, DC: NOCA.

National Commission for Health Education Credentialing, Inc. (1996). *A Competency-based framework for professional development of certified health education specialists.* Allentown, PA: Author.

National Commission for Health Education Credentialing, Society for Public Health Education, & American Association for Health Education. (2006). *A competency-based framework for health educators - 2006.* Whitehall, PA: Author.

National Commission for Health Education Credentialing, Inc. (2007). *The health education specialist: A study guide for professional competence* (5th ed.). Whitehall, PA: Author.

National Commission for Health Education Credentialing, Inc. (2008a). *CHES exam receives "Gold Standard" NCCA accreditation.* Retrieved from http://www.nchec.org/news/what/#BM_NCH-MR-TAB2-30

National Commission for Health Education Credentialing, Inc. (2008b). Competencies update project. Retrieved from: http://www.nchec.org/credentialing/docs/nch-mr-tab3-111.htm

National Commission for Health Education Credentialing, Inc. (2009). *NCHEC board of commissioners pass policy statement regarding the advance credential.* Retrieved from http://www.nchec.org/_files/_items/nch-mr-tab2-163/docs/mches%20press%20 release%20%205-29-09.pdf

National Task Force on the Preparation & Practice of Health Education Specialists. (1985). *A framework for the development of competency-based curricula for entry-level health education specialists.* New York, NY: National Commission for Health Education Credentialing, Inc.

Neutens, J. (1984). Professional Competencies of the Health Educator. In L. Rubinson & W.Alles (Eds.), *Health Education Foundations for the Future.* Prospect Heights, IL: Waveland Press.

Raymond, M. R. (2002). A practical guide to practice analysis for credentialing examinations. *Educational Measurement: Issues and Practice*, 21(3), 25-37.

Society for Public Health Education, & American Association for Health Education (1997). *Standards for the preparation of graduate-level health educators.* Washington, DC: Author.

Society for Public Health Education, & American Association for Health Education. (2007). *SOPHE/AAHE baccalaureate program approval committee manual: Criteria, process, & procedures for quality assurance in community health education.* Washington, DC: Author.

Tabachnick, B.G., & Fidell, L.S. (2005). *Using multivariate statistics* (5th ed.). Boston, MA: Allyn and Bacon.

Taub, A., Birch, D. A., Auld, M. E., Lysoby, L., & Rasar King, L. (2009). Strengthening quality assurance in health education: Recent milestones and future directions. *Health Promotion Practice*, 10, 192-200.

United States Department of Health, Education and Welfare, Health Resources Administration, Bureau of Health Manpower. (1978). *Preparation and practice of community, patient, and school health educators: Proceedings of the workshop on commonalities and differences.* Washington, DC: Division of Allied Health Professions.

Woodhouse, L., Auld, M. E., Miner, K., Alley, K. B., Lysoby, L., & Livingood, W. (2010) Crosswalking public health and health education competencies: Implications for professional preparation and practice. *Journal of Public Health Management and Practice*, 16(3), E20-8.

Woudenberg, F. (1991). An evaluation of Delphi. *Technological Forecasting and Social Change*, 40(2), 131-150.

REFERENCES

Appendices

Glossary

The glossary explains terms used in this document. These definitions are not all-inclusive but are intended to convey the meaning of terms within the context of this document.

Advanced-level 1 – The practice level of a health education specialist with a baccalaureate or a master's degree and five or more years of experience in the field of health education.

Advanced-level 2 – The practice level of a health education specialist with a doctoral degree and five or more years of experience in the field of health education.

Area of Responsibility – One of the major categories of performance expectations of a proficient health education practitioner. The Areas of Responsibility define the scope of practice (SOPHE & AAHE, 1997).

Certified Health Education Specialist (CHES) – An individual who has met academic eligibility in health education, passed a written examination administered by the National Commission for Health Education Credentialing, Inc., and has an ongoing commitment to continuing education.

Master Certified Health Education Specialist (MCHES) – An individual who has met academic eligibility in health education and is practicing at the advanced-level in the field, passed a written examination administered by the National Commission for Health Education Credentialing, Inc., and has an ongoing commitment to continuing education.

Credentialing – An umbrella term referring to the various means employed to designate that individuals or organizations have met or exceeded established standards. These standards may include certification, registration, or licensure of individuals or accreditation of organizations. Health education has chosen certification as the method of individual credentialing for the profession (NCHEC, n.d.).

Coalition – An alliance, often temporary, that allows two or more groups or organizations to promote a common cause (AAHE, NCHEC, & SOPHE, 1999).

Competency – A broadly defined skill or ability, adequate performance of which is expected of the health educator. Mastery of a competency is dependent upon achievement of clusters of simpler but essential related skills or abilities (NCHEC, 1990).

Entry-level – The practice level of a health education specialist with a baccalaureate or master degree and less than five years of experience in the field of health education.

Health education – Any combination of planned learning experiences based on sound theories that provide individuals, groups, and communities the opportunity to acquire the information and skills needed to make quality health decisions (Joint Committee on Health Education and Promotion Terminology, 2001).

Health education specialist (formerly "health educator") – A professionally prepared individual who serves in a variety of roles and is specifically trained to use appropriate educational strategies and methods to facilitate the development of policies, procedures, interventions, and systems conducive to the health of individuals, groups, and communities (Joint Committee on Health Education and Promotion Terminology, 2001).

Health literacy – The capacity of an individual to obtain, interpret, and understand basic health information and services and the competence to use such information and services in ways that are health enhancing (Joint Committee on Health Education and Promotion Terminology, 2001).

Profession – A group of individuals with similar educational preparation who come together for a common occupational goal and that usually exhibits the following characteristics: (1) provides a unique and essential service; (2) requires of its members an extensive period of preparation; (3) has a theoretical base underlying its practice; (4) has a system of internal controls, including a code of ethics that tends to regulate the behavior of its members; (5) has a culture peculiar to the profession; 6) is sanctioned by the community; and (7) has an occupational association representative of and able to speak on behalf of all members of the profession (Neutens, 1984).

Professional development – Planned learning activities designed to maintain and enhance one's competence in health education following a previously attained level of professional preparation (Joint Committee on Health Education and Promotion Terminology, 2001).

Professional preparation – An undergraduate or graduate course of study that includes career-related experiences offered through an accredited college or university, which is designed to prepare individuals to practice competently in the health education field (Joint Committee on Health Education and Promotion Terminology, 2001).

Standard – The predetermined level of performance at which a criterion will be considered met. If a desired condition or characteristic (e.g., curricular content that assures development of specific health education competencies) is the criterion, the standard then expresses the minimum acceptable content that will satisfy the expectation (AAHE, NCHEC, & SOPHE, 1999).

APPENDIX A

Comparison of the Areas of Responsibility, Competencies, and Sub-competencies of the CUP Model and the HEJA 2010 Model

Adoption of the HEJA 2010 Model as the framework for certification, professional preparation, and professional development has generated the need to adapt criteria and materials used for these three purposes. To help facilitate these adaptations, a subcommittee from the NCHEC Division Board for Certification of Health Education compared the Areas of Responsibility, Competencies, and Sub-competencies of the CUP Model and the HEJA 2010 Model. Tables B.1 and B.2 illustrate comparison results.

Table B.1 can be used to identify specific Competencies and Sub-competencies in the Old (CUP) model that were re-assigned and/or revised and integrated into a different Area and/or Competency in the New (HEJA 2010) Model. For example, the first Competency in the CUP Model under *Area of Responsibility I was Competency A: Access existing health-related data* (see column marked "CUP"). In the HEJA 2010 model, that Competency is now *Competency 1.2* (see "HEJA" column). As can be noted in the Table, *Sub-competency I.A.E.1: Identify diverse health-related databases* in the Cup Model became *Sub-competency 1.2.1: Identify sources of data related to health* in the HEJA 2010 Model.

Though the comparison results are useful for the realignment of items on the certification exam and for adjusting curricula in professional preparation programs, it should be noted that the comparison was based on specific wording, not on intent of use. This perspective is particularly important when interpreting the word "Loss" assigned to some Sub-competencies in Table B.1, which only means that a Sub-competency with specific or highly similar wording does not exist in the HEJA 2010 Model. However, many of these Sub-competencies were subsumed within the context of other Sub-competencies in the HEJA 2010 Model.

The format of Table B.2 is similar to that of Table B.1; however, Table B.2 contains the Areas of Responsibility, Competencies, and Sub-competencies of the New (HEJA 2010) Model. To the right of most Competencies and Sub-competencies in the New model (see "HEJA" columns) is the lettered label for similarly-worded Competencies or Sub-competencies in the Old model (see "CUP" columns). For some, the word "New" is listed in that column to denote that no Competency or Sub-competency containing that specific wording existed in the Old model; however, the caution provided for interpreting the word "Loss" in Table B.1 should also be used in interpreting the word "New" in Table B.2. Identification of a Sub-competency as 'new' merely indicates that it did not exist as worded in the previous model.

The seasoned health education specialist will likely note that the HEJA 2010 Model contains most of the Competencies and Sub-competencies of the CUP Model, along with some additional components that reflect the contemporary practice of health education specialists at the entry-, advanced 1-, and advanced 2-levels. One of the benefits of the HEJA 2010 Model is that most Sub-competencies emerged in straightforward language with one clear function that should facilitate clear interpretation and effective application of the model.

Table B.1

Comparison of CUP Model (old) and HEJA 2010 Model (new): The Cup Model (old) perspective

		Entry (Baccalaureate/Master's and Less Than 5 Years' Experience)		Advanced 1 (Baccalaureate/Master's and 5 Years' Experience or More)		Advanced 2 (Doctorate and 5 Years' Experience or More)	
CUP	HEJA	CUP	HEJA	CUP	HEJA	CUP	HEJA
Area of Responsibility I: Assess Individual and Community Needs for Health Education							
I. Competency A: Access existing health-related data	1.2	I.A.E.1. Identify diverse health-related databases	1.2.1				
		I.A.E.2. Use computerized sources of health-related information	Loss			I.A.A2.1. Critique sources of health information	1.2.2
		I.A.E.3. Determine the compatibility of data from different data sources	Loss				
		I.A.E.4. Select valid sources of information about health needs and interests	1.2.3				
I. Competency B: Collect health-related data	1.3	I.B.E.1. Use appropriate data-gathering instruments	1.3.6				
		I.B.E.2. Apply survey techniques to acquire health data	1.3.6				
		I.B.E.3. Conduct health-related needs assessments	Loss				
		I.B.E.4. Implement appropriate measures to assess capacity for improving health status	Loss				
I. Competency C: Distinguish between behaviors that foster or hinder well-being	1.4	I.C.E.1. Identify diverse factors that influence health behaviors	1.4.1	I.C.A1.1. Explain the role of experiences in shaping patterns of health behavior	Loss		

CUP	HEJA	Entry (Baccalaureate/Master's and Less Than 5 Years' Experience) CUP	HEJA	Advanced 1 (Baccalaureate/Master's and 5 Years' Experience or More) CUP	HEJA	Advanced 2 (Doctorate and 5 Years' Experience or More) CUP	HEJA
I. Competency D: Determine factors that influence learning	1.5	I.C.E.2. Identify behaviors that tend to promote or compromise health	1.4.3	I.D.A1.1. Assess learning literacy I.D.A1.2. Assess learning styles	1.5.1	I.D.A2.1. Assess the learning environment	1.5.1
I. Competency E: Identify factors that foster or hinder the process of health education	1.6	I.E.E.1. Determine the extent of available health education services	1.6.1	I.E.A1.1. Assess the environmental and political climate (e.g., organizational, community, state, and national) regarding conditions that advance or inhibit program goals	1.6.4	I.E.A2.1. Investigate social forces causing opposing viewpoints regarding health education needs and concerns	Loss
		I.E.E.2. Identify gaps and overlaps in the provision of collaborative health services	1.2.4				
I. Competency F: Infer needs for health education from obtained data	1.7	I.F.E.1. Analyze needs assessment data	1.7.1	I.F.A1.1. Determine priorities for health education	1.7.3	I.F.A2.1. Predict future health education needs based upon societal changes	Loss
Area of Responsibility II: Plan Health Education Strategies, Interventions, and Programs							
II. Competency A: Involve people and organizations in program planning	2.1	II.A.E.1. Identify populations for health education programs	2.1.2	II.A.A1.1. Involve participants in planning health education programs	5.3.3		
		II.A.E.2. Elicit input from those who will affect, or be affected by, the program	2.1.5				
		II.A.E.3. Obtain commitments from individuals who will be involved in the program	2.1.6				
		II.A.E.4. Develop plans for promoting collaborative efforts among health agencies and organizations with mutual interests	2.1.4				

CUP	HEJA	Entry (Baccalaureate/Master's and Less Than 5 Years' Experience)		Advanced 1 (Baccalaureate/Master's and 5 Years' Experience or More)		Advanced 2 (Doctorate and 5 Years' Experience or More)	
		CUP	HEJA	CUP	HEJA	CUP	HEJA
II. Competency B: Incorporate data analysis and principles of community organization	Loss	II.B.E.1. Use research results when planning programs	Loss	II.B.A1.1. Incorporate results of needs assessment into the planning process	2.2.1		
		II.B.E.2. Apply principles of community organization when planning programs	2.1.1				
		II.B.E.3. Suggest approaches for integrating health education within existing health programs	Loss				
		II.B.E.4. Communicate need for the program to those who will be involved	2.1.3				
II. Competency C: Formulate appropriate and measurable program objectives	2.2	II.C.E.1. Design developmentally appropriate interventions	2.3	II.C.A1.1. Establish criteria for health education program objectives	2.2.5	II.C.A2.1. Develop subordinate measurable objectives as needed for instruction	Loss
				II.C.A1.2. Develop program objectives based upon identified needs	2.2.5		
				II.C.A1.3. Appraise appropriateness of resources and materials relative to given objectives	Loss	II.C.A2.2. Evaluate the efficacy of various methods to achieve objectives	2.3.1
				II.C.A1.4. Revise program objectives as necessitated by changing needs	Loss		
II. Competency D: Develop a logical scope and sequence plan for health education practice	2.4	II.D.E.1. Determine the range of health information necessary for a given program of instruction	2.4.1	II.D.A1.1. Organize the subject areas comprising the scope of a program in logical sequence	2.4.4	II.D.A2.1. Incorporate theory-based foundations in planning health education programs	Loss

CUP	HEJA	Entry (Baccalaureate/Master's and Less Than 5 Years' Experience)		Advanced 1 (Baccalaureate/Master's and 5 Years' Experience or More)		Advanced 2 (Doctorate and 5 Years' Experience or More)	
		CUP	HEJA	CUP	HEJA	CUP	HEJA
II. Competency E: Design strategies, interventions, and programs consistent with specified objectives	2.3	II.D.E.2. Select references relevant to health education issues or programs		II.D.A1.2. Analyze the process for integrating health education into other programs	2.4.2		2.4.6
				II.E.A1.1. Plan a sequence of learning opportunities that reinforce mastery of preceding objectives		II.E.A2.1. Formulate a variety of educational methods	Loss
				II.E.A1.2. Select strategies best suited to achieve objectives in a given setting		II.E.A2.2. Match proposed learning activities with stated program objectives	Loss
						II.E.A2.3. Select appropriate theory-based strategies in health program planning	Loss
II. Competency F: Select appropriate strategies to meet objectives	2.3	II.F.E.1. Analyze technologies, methods, and media for their acceptability to diverse groups	Loss	II.F.A1.1. Plan training and instructional programs for diverse populations	Loss	II.F.A2.1. Select educational materials consistent with accepted theory	Loss
		II.F.E.2. Match health education services to proposed program activities	Loss	II.F.A1.2. Incorporate communication strategies into program planning	Loss		
II. Competency G: Assess factors that affect implementation	2.5	II.G.E.1. Determine the availability of information and resources needed to implement health education programs for a given audience	Loss	II.G.A1.1. Analyze factors (e.g., learner characteristics, legal aspects, feasibility) that influence choices among implementation methods	2.5.2		
		II.G.E.2. Identify barriers to the implementation of health education programs	2.5.1	II.G.A1.2. Select implementation strategies based upon research results	Loss		

Area of Responsibility III: Implement Health Education Strategies, Interventions, and Programs

CUP	HEJA	Entry (Baccalaureate/Master's and Less Than 5 Years' Experience)		Advanced 1 (Baccalaureate/Master's and 5 Years' Experience or More)		Advanced 2 (Doctorate and 5 Years' Experience or More)	
		CUP	HEJA	CUP	HEJA	CUP	HEJA
III. Competency A: Initiate a plan of action	3.1	III.A.E.1. Use community organization principles to facilitate change conducive to health	2.1.1				
		III.A.E.2. Pretest learners to determine baseline data relative to proposed program objectives	3.1.2	III.A.A1.1. Apply individual or group process methods as appropriate to given learning situations	2.1.6		
		III.A.E.3. Deliver educational programs to diverse populations	3.1.7				
		III.A.E.4. Facilitate groups	Loss				
III. Competency B: Demonstrate a variety of skills in delivering strategies, interventions, and programs	Loss	III.B.E.1. Use instructional technology effectively	Loss	III.B.A1.1. Select methods that best facilitate achievement of program objectives	Loss	III.B.A2.1. Use a variety of educational methods	3.1.4
		III.B.E.2. Apply implementation strategies	Loss	III.B.A1.2. Apply technologies that will contribute to program objectives	Loss		
III. Competency C: Use a variety of methods to implement strategies, interventions, and programs	Loss	III.C.E.1. Use the Code of Ethics in professional practice	1.3.7 2.3.4 3.2.5 4.1.14 4.3.6 5.3.6 5.4.8 6.3.8	III.C.A1.1. Employ appropriate strategies when dealing with controversial health issues	Loss		
		III.C.E.2. Apply theoretical and conceptual models from health education and related disciplines to improve program delivery	Loss				

Competency	CUP	HEJA	Entry (Baccalaureate/Master's and Less Than 5 Years' Experience) CUP	Entry HEJA	Advanced 1 (Baccalaureate/Master's and 5 Years' Experience or More) CUP	Advanced 1 HEJA	Advanced 2 (Doctorate and 5 Years' Experience or More) CUP	Advanced 2 HEJA
III. Competency D: Conduct training programs		3.3	III.C.E.3. Demonstrate skills needed to develop capacity for improving health status	Loss	III.D.A1.1. Demonstrate a wide range of strategies for conducting training programs	3.3.5	III.D.A2.1. Use instructional resources that meet a variety of training needs	Loss
			III.C.E.4. Incorporate demographically and culturally sensitive techniques when promoting programs	Loss				
			III.C.E.5. Implement intervention strategies to facilitate health-related change	Loss				

Area of Responsibility IV: Conduct Evaluation and Research Related to Health Education

Competency	CUP	HEJA	Entry (Baccalaureate/Master's and Less Than 5 Years' Experience) CUP	Entry HEJA	Advanced 1 (Baccalaureate/Master's and 5 Years' Experience or More) CUP	Advanced 1 HEJA	Advanced 2 (Doctorate and 5 Years' Experience or More) CUP	Advanced 2 HEJA
IV. Competency A: Develop plans for evaluation and research		4.1	IV.A.E.1. Synthesize information presented in the literature	4.1.5	IV.A.A1.1. Develop an inventory of existing valid and reliable tests and survey instruments	4.1.8	IV.A.A2.1. Assess the merits and limitations of qualitative and quantitative methods	4.1.6
			IV.A.E.2. Evaluate research designs, methods, and findings presented in the literature	4.1.4				
IV. Competency B: Review research and evaluation procedures		Loss	IV.B.E.1. Evaluate data-gathering instruments and processes	4.1.9	IV.B.A1.1. Identify standards of performance to be applied as criteria of effectiveness	Loss	IV.B.A2.1. Establish a realistic scope of evaluation efforts	Loss
			IV.B.E.2. Develop methods to evaluate factors that influence shifts in health status	Loss	IV.B.A1.2. Identify methods to evaluate factors that influence shifts in health status	Loss	IV.B.A2.2. Select appropriate qualitative and/or quantitative evaluation design	Loss
					IV.B.A1.3. Select appropriate methods for evaluating program effectiveness	Loss		

CUP	HEJA	Entry (Baccalaureate/Master's and Less Than 5 Years' Experience)		Advanced 1 (Baccalaureate/Master's and 5 Years' Experience or More)		Advanced 2 (Doctorate and 5 Years' Experience or More)	
		CUP	HEJA	CUP	HEJA	CUP	HEJA
IV. Competency C: Design data collection instruments	4.2	IV.C.E.1. Develop valid and reliable evaluation instruments	4.2.4 4.2.5				
		IV.C.E.2. Develop appropriate data-gathering instruments	Loss				
IV. Competency D: Carry out evaluation and research plans	Loss	IV.D.E.1. Use appropriate research methods and designs in health education practice	Loss	IV.D.A1.1. Assess the relevance of existing program objectives to current needs	Loss	IV.D.A2.1. Apply appropriate evaluation technology	Loss
		IV.D.E.2. Use data collection methods appropriate for measuring stated objectives	Loss				
		IV.D.E.3. Implement appropriate qualitative and quantitative evaluation techniques	Loss			IV.D.A2.2. Analyze evaluation data	
		IV.D.E.4. Implement methods to evaluate factors that influence shifts in health status	Loss				
IV. Competency E: Interpret results from evaluation and research	4.4	IV.E.E.1. Analyze evaluation data	4.3.5 4.3.4 4.3.3	IV.E.A1.1. Compare program activities with the stated program objectives	Loss	IV.E.A2.1. Determine the achievement of objectives by applying criteria to evaluation results	Loss
		IV.E.E.2. Analyze research data	4.3.5 4.3.4 4.3.3				
		IV.E.E.3. Compare evaluation results to other findings	4.4.2	IV.E.A1.2. Develop recommendations based upon evaluation results	4.4.5	IV.E.A2.2. Communicate evaluation results using easily understood terms	4.5.1
		IV.E.E.4. Report effectiveness of programs in achieving proposed objectives	Loss				
IV. Competency F: Infer implications from findings for future health-related activities	Loss			IV.F.A1.1. Suggest strategies for implementing recommendations that result from evaluation	Loss	IV.F.A2.1. Propose possible explanations for evaluation findings	4.4.3
				IV.F.A1.2. Apply evaluation findings to refine and maintain programs			

Area of Responsibility V: Administer Health Education Strategies, Interventions, and Programs

		Entry (Baccalaureate/Master's and Less Than 5 Years' Experience)		Advanced 1 (Baccalaureate/Master's and 5 Years' Experience or More)		Advanced 2 (Doctorate and 5 Years' Experience or More)	
CUP	HEJA	CUP	HEJA	CUP	HEJA	CUP	HEJA
V. Competency A: Exercise organizational leadership	5.3	V.A.E.1. Conduct strategic planning	5.3.1	V.A.A1.1. Develop strategies to reinforce or change organizational culture to achieve program goals	5.3.4	V.A.A2.1. Facilitate administration of the evaluation plan	Loss
		V.A.E.2. Analyze the organization's culture in relationship to program goals	5.3.6	V.A.A1.2. Ensure that program activities comply with existing laws and regulations	5.3.5		
		V.A.E.3. Promote cooperation and feedback among personnel related to the program	Loss	V.A.A1.3. Develop budgets to support program requirements	5.1.3		
V. Competency B: Secure fiscal resources	5.1			V.B.A1.1. Manage program budgets.	5.1.4	V.B.A2.1. Prepare proposals to obtain fiscal resources	5.1.2
V. Competency C: Manage human resources	5.4	V.C.E.1. Develop volunteer opportunities	5.4.1	V.C.A1.1. Demonstrate leadership in managing human resources	5.4.2		
				V.C.A1.2. Apply human resource policies consistent with relevant laws and regulations	5.4.3		
				V.C.A1.3. Identify qualifications of personnel needed for programs	5.4.4		
				V.C.A1.4. Facilitate staff development	5.4.9 5.4.10		
				V.C.A1.5. Apply appropriate methods of conflict reduction	5.4.6		

		Entry *(Baccalaureate/Master's and Less Than 5 Years' Experience)*		Advanced 1 *(Baccalaureate/Master's and 5 Years' Experience or More)*		Advanced 2 *(Doctorate and 5 Years' Experience or More)*	
CUP	HEJA	**CUP**	HEJA	**CUP**	HEJA	**CUP**	HEJA
V. Competency D: Obtain acceptance and support for programs	5.2			V.D.A1.1. Use concepts and theories of public relations and communications to obtain program support	5.2.1	V.D.A2.1. Provide support for individuals who deliver professional development courses	5.2.5
				V.D.A1.2. Facilitate cooperation among personnel responsible for health education programs	5.2.2		
Area of Responsibility VI: Serve as a Health Education Resource Person							
VI. Competency A: Use health-related information resources	Loss	VI.A.E.1. Match information needs with the appropriate retrieval systems	6.1.1 6.1.2				
		VI.A.E.2. Select a data system commensurate with program needs	Loss				
		VI.A.E.3. Determine the relevance of various computerized health information resources	6.1.3				
		VI.A.E.4. Access health information resources	Loss				
		VI.A.E.5. Employ electronic technology for retrieving references	Loss				
VI. Competency B: Respond to requests for health information	Loss	VI.B.E.1. Identify information sources needed to satisfy a request	6.3.2				
		VI.B.E.2. Refer requesters to valid sources of health information	Loss				
VI. Competency C: Select resource materials for dissemination	Loss	VI.C.E.1. Evaluate applicability of resource materials for given audience	Loss				

VI. Competency D: Establish consultative relationships	HEJA	Entry (Baccalaureate/Master's and Less Than 5 Years' Experience)		Advanced 1 (Baccalaureate/Master's and 5 Years' Experience or More)		Advanced 2 (Doctorate and 5 Years' Experience or More)	
		CUP	HEJA	CUP	HEJA	CUP	HEJA
		VI.C.E.2. Apply various processes to acquire resource materials	Loss				
		VI.C.E.3. Assemble educational material of value to the health of individuals and community groups	Loss				
		VI.D.E.1. Analyze parameters of effective consultative relationships	6.3.3				
	6.3	VI.D.E.2. Analyze the role of the health educator as a liaison between program staff and outside groups and organizations	Loss				
		VI.D.E.3. Act as a liaison among consumer groups, individuals, and health care provider organizations	Loss				
		VI.D.E.4. Apply networking skills to develop and maintain consultative relationships	Loss			VI.D.A2.1. Describe consulting skills needed by health educators	Loss
		VI.D.E.5. Facilitate collaborative training efforts among health agencies and organizations	6.3.6				

Area of Responsibility VII: Communicate and Advocate for Health and Health Education

	Entry (Baccalaureate/Master's and Less Than 5 Years' Experience) CUP	Entry HEJA	Advanced 1 (Baccalaureate/Master's and 5 Years' Experience or More) CUP	Advanced 1 HEJA	Advanced 2 (Doctorate and 5 Years' Experience or More) CUP	Advanced 2 HEJA
VII. Competency A: Analyze and respond to current and future needs in health education	VII.A.E.1. Analyze factors (e.g, social, cultural, demographic, and political) that influence decision-makers	New / 7.1.4	VII.A.A1.1. Respond to challenges facing health education programs	Loss	VII.A.A2.1. Analyze the interrelationships among ethics, values, and behavior	Loss
			VII.A.A1.2. Implement strategies for advocacy initiatives	7.4.2	VII.A.A2.2. Relate health education issues to larger social issues	Loss
			VII.A.A1.3. Use evaluation data to advocate for health education programs	7.4.5		
VII. Competency B: Apply a variety of communication methods and techniques	VII.B.E.1. Assess the appropriateness of language in health education messages	7.2 / Loss				
	VII.B.E.2. Compare different methods of distributing educational materials	Loss				
	VII.B.E.3. Respond to public input regarding health education information	Loss				
	VII.B.E.4. Use culturally sensitive communication methods and techniques	Loss				
	VII.B.E.5. Use appropriate techniques when communicating health and health education information	7.2.4				
	VII.B.E.6. Use oral, electronic, and written techniques for communicating health education information	7.3.2				

CUP	HEJA	Entry (Baccalaureate/Master's and Less Than 5 Years' Experience)		Advanced 1 (Baccalaureate/Master's and 5 Years' Experience or More)		Advanced 2 (Doctorate and 5 Years' Experience or More)	
		CUP	HEJA	CUP	HEJA	CUP	HEJA
VII. Competency C: Promote the health education profession individually and collectively	7.6	VII.B.E.7. Demonstrate proficiency in communicating health information and health education needs	Loss				
		VII.C.E.1. Develop a personal plan for professional growth	7.6.1				
						VII.C.A2.1. Describe the state-of-the-art of health education practice	7.6.2
						VII.C.A2.2. Explain the major responsibilities of the health educator in the practice of health education	7.6.3
						VII.C.A2.3. Explain the role of health education associations in advancing the profession	7.6.4
						VII.C.A2.4. Explain the benefits of participating in professional organizations	7.6.5
VII. Competency D: Influence health policy to promote health	7.5.	VII.D.E.1. Identify the significance and implications of health care providers' messages to consumers	Loss	VII.D.A1.1. Use research results to develop health policy	7.5.4	VII.D.A2.1. Describe how research results influence health policy	Loss
						VII.D.A2.2. Use evaluation findings in policy analysis and development	7.5.1

APPENDIX B

Table B.2

Comparison of CUP Model (old) and HEJA 2010 Model (new): The HEJA 2010 Model (new) perspective

Area of Responsibility		Entry (Baccalaureate/Master's and Less Than 5 Years' Experience)		Advanced 1 (Baccalaureate/Master's and 5 Years' Experience or More)		Advanced 2 (Doctorate and 5 Years' Experience or More)	
HEJA	CUP	**HEJA**	CUP	**HEJA**	CUP	**HEJA**	CUP
Area of Responsibility 1: Assess Needs, Assets, and Capacity for Health Education							
1.1 Plan assessment process	New	1.1.1 Identify existing and needed resources to conduct assessments	New	1.1.2 Identify stakeholders to participate in the assessment process	New		
		1.1.3 Apply theories and models to develop assessment strategies	New				
		1.1.4 Develop plans for data collection, analysis, and interpretation	New	1.1.5 Engage stakeholders to participate in the assessment process	New		
		1.1.6. Integrate research designs, methods, and instruments into assessment plans	New				
1.2 Access existing information and data related to health	I.A.	1.2.1 Identify sources of data related to health	I.A.E.1				
		1.2.2 Critique sources of health information using theory and evidence from the literature	I.A.A2.1				
		1.2.3 Select valid sources of information about health	I.A.E.4				
		1.2.4 Identify gaps in data using theories and assessment models	I.E.E.2				
		1.2.5 Establish collaborative relationships and agreements that facilitate access to data	New				
		1.2.6 Conduct searches of existing databases for specific health-related data	I.B.E.1 I.B.E.2				

HEJA	CUP	Entry (Baccalaureate/Master's and Less Than 5 Years' Experience) HEJA	Entry CUP	Advanced 1 (Baccalaureate/Master's and 5 Years' Experience or More) HEJA	Advanced 1 CUP	Advanced 2 (Doctorate and 5 Years' Experience or More) HEJA	Advanced 2 CUP
1.3 Collect quantitative and/or qualitative data related to health	I.B.	1.3.1 Collect primary and/or secondary data	New				
		1.3.2 Integrate primary data with secondary data	New				
		1.3.3 Identify data collection instruments and methods	New				
		1.3.4 Develop data collection instruments and methods	New				
		1.3.5 Train personnel and stakeholders regarding data collection	New				
		1.3.6 Use data collection instruments and methods	I.B.E.1 I.B.E.2				
		1.3.7 Employ ethical standards when collecting data	III.C.E.1				
1.4 Examine relationships among behavioral, environmental and genetic factors that enhance or compromise health	I.C.	1.4.1 Identify factors that influence health behaviors	I.C.E.1				
		1.4.2 Analyze factors that influence health behaviors	New				
		1.4.3 Identify factors that enhance or compromise health	I.C.E.2				
		1.4.4 Analyze factors that enhance or compromise health	New				
1.5 Examine factors that influence the learning process	I.D.	1.5.1 Identify factors that foster or hinder the learning process	I.D.A1.1 I.D.A1.2 I.D.A2.1			1.5.2 Analyze factors that foster or hinder the learning process	I.D.A1.1 I.D.A1.2 I.D.A2.1
		1.5.3 Identify factors that foster or hinder attitudes and beliefs	New				

HEJA	CUP	Entry (Baccalaureate/Master's and Less Than 5 Years' Experience) HEJA	Entry CUP	Advanced 1 (Baccalaureate/Master's and 5 Years' Experience or More) HEJA	Advanced 1 CUP	Advanced 2 (Doctorate and 5 Years' Experience or More) HEJA	Advanced 2 CUP
		1.5.4 Analyze factors that foster or hinder attitudes and beliefs	New			1.5.5 Identify factors that foster or hinder skill building	I.D.A1.1 I.D.A1.2 I.D.A2.1
						1.5.6 Analyze factors that foster or hinder skill building	I.D.A1.1 I.D.A1.2 I.D.A2.1
1.6 Examine factors that enhance or compromise the process of health education	I.E.	1.6.1 Determine the extent of available health education programs, interventions, and policies	I.E.E1				
		1.6.2 Assess the quality of available health education programs, interventions, and policies	New				
		1.6.3 Identify existing and potential partners for the provision of health education	New				
		1.6.4 Assess social, environmental, and political conditions that may impact health education	I.E.A1.1				
		1.6.5 Analyze the capacity for developing needed health education	New				
		1.6.6 Assess the need for resources to foster health education	New				
1.7 Infer needs for health education based on assessment findings	I.F.	1.7.1 Analyze assessment findings	I.F.E.1.			1.7.2 Synthesize assessment findings	New
		1.7.3 Prioritize health education needs	I.F.A1.1.				
		1.7.4 Identify emerging health education needs	New				

	HEJA	CUP	Entry (Baccalaureate/Master's and Less Than 5 Years' Experience) HEJA	Entry CUP	Advanced 1 (Baccalaureate/Master's and 5 Years' Experience or More) HEJA	Advanced 1 CUP	Advanced 2 (Doctorate and 5 Years' Experience or More) HEJA	Advanced 2 CUP
			1.7.5 Report assessment findings	New				
Area of Responsibility II: Plan Health Education								
2.1 Involve priority populations and other stakeholders in the planning process		II.A.	2.1.1 Incorporate principles of community organization	II.B.E.2				
			2.1.2 Identify priority populations and other stakeholders	II.A.E.1				
			2.1.3 Communicate need for health education to priority populations and other stakeholders	II.B.E.4				
			2.1.4 Develop collaborative efforts among priority populations and other stakeholders	II.A.E.4				
			2.1.5 Elicit input from priority populations and other stakeholders	II.A.E.2				
			2.1.6 Obtain commitments from priority populations and other stakeholders	II.A.E.3				
2.2 Develop goals and objectives		II.C	2.2.2 Identify desired outcomes utilizing the needs assessment results	New	2.2.1 Use assessment results to inform the planning process	II.B.A.1.1	2.2.3 Select planning model(s) for health education	New
					2.2.4 Develop goal statements	New		
					2.2.5 Formulate specific, measurable, attainable,	II.C.A1.1 II.C.A.1.2		

HEJA	CUP	Entry (Baccalaureate/Master's and Less Than 5 Years' Experience) HEJA	CUP	Advanced 1 (Baccalaureate/Master's and 5 Years' Experience or More) HEJA	CUP	Advanced 2 (Doctorate and 5 Years' Experience or More) HEJA	CUP
		2.2.6 Assess resources needed to achieve objectives	New	realistic, and time-sensitive objectives			
2.3 Select or design strategies and interventions	II.E II.F	2.3.2 Design theory-based strategies and interventions to achieve stated objectives	New				
		2.3.4 Comply with legal and ethical principles in designing strategies and interventions	III.C.E.1	2.3.3 Select a variety of strategies and interventions to achieve stated objectives	New	2.3.1 Assess efficacy of various strategies to ensure consistency with objectives	II.C.A.2.2
		2.3.5 Apply principles of cultural competence in selecting and designing strategies and interventions	New				
		2.3.6 Pilot test strategies and interventions	New				
2.4 Develop a scope and sequence for the delivery of health education	II.D	2.4.1 Determine the range of health education needed to achieve goals and objectives	II.D.E.1				
		2.4.2 Select resources required to implement health education	II.D.E.2	2.4.4 Organize health education into a logical sequence	II.D.A1.1		
		2.4.3 Use logic models to guide the planning process	New	2.4.5 Develop a timeline for the delivery of health education	New		
		2.4.6 Analyze the opportunity for integrating health education into other programs	II.D.A1.2				

HEJA	CUP	Entry (Baccalaureate/Master's and Less Than 5 Years' Experience)		Advanced 1 (Baccalaureate/Master's and 5 Years' Experience or More)		Advanced 2 (Doctorate and 5 Years' Experience or More)	
		HEJA	CUP	HEJA	CUP	HEJA	CUP
		2.4.7 Develop a process for integrating health education into other programs	New				
2.5 Address factors that affect implementation	II.G.	2.5.1 Identify factors that foster or hinder implementation	II.G.E.2				
		2.5.2 Analyze factors that foster or hinder implementation	II.G.A1.1				
		2.5.3 Use findings of pilot to refine implementation plans as needed	New				
		2.5.4 Develop a conducive learning environment	New				
Area of Responsibility III: Implement Health Education							
3.1 Implement a plan of action	III.A.	3.1.1 Assess readiness for implementation	New				
		3.1.2 Collect baseline data	II.A.E.2				
		3.1.3 Use strategies to ensure cultural competence in implementing health education plans	New				
		3.1.4 Use a variety of strategies to deliver a plan of action	III.B.A2.1				
		3.1.5 Promote plan of action	New				
		3.1.6 Apply theories and models of implementation	III.A.A1.1				
		3.1.7 Launch plan of action	III.A.E.3				
3.2 Monitor implementation of health education	New	3.2.1 Monitor progress in accordance with timeline	New				
		3.2.2 Assess progress in achieving objectives	New				

		Entry (Baccalaureate/Master's and Less Than 5 Years' Experience)		Advanced 1 (Baccalaureate/Master's and 5 Years' Experience or More)		Advanced 2 (Doctorate and 5 Years' Experience or More)	
HEJA	**CUP**	**HEJA**	**CUP**	**HEJA**	**CUP**	**HEJA**	**CUP**
		3.2.3 Modify plan of action as needed	New				
		3.2.4 Monitor use of resources	New				
		3.2.5 Monitor compliance with legal and ethical principles	III.C.E.1				
				3.3.2 Identify training needs	New		
3.3 Train individuals involved in implementation of health education	III.D.	3.3.1 Select training participants needed for implementation	New	3.3.3 Develop training objectives	New		
		3.3.5 Demonstrate a wide range of training strategies	III.D.A1.1	3.3.4 Create training using best practices	New		
		3.3.6 Deliver training	New	3.3.7 Evaluate training	New		
				3.3.8 Use evaluation findings to plan future training	New		

Area of Responsibility IV: Conduct Evaluation and Research Related to Health Education

		Entry HEJA	Entry CUP			Advanced 2 HEJA	Advanced 2 CUP
						4.1.1 Create purpose statement	New
4.1 Develop evaluation/research plan	IV.4.	4.1.3 Assess feasibility of conducting evaluation/research	New			4.1.2 Develop evaluation/research questions	New
		4.1.4 Critique evaluation and research methods and findings found in the related literature	IV.A.E.2				
		4.1.5 Synthesize information found in the literature	IV.A.E.1				

HEJA	CUP	Entry (Baccalaureate/Master's and Less Than 5 Years' Experience) HEJA	Entry CUP	Advanced 1 (Baccalaureate/Master's and 5 Years' Experience or More) HEJA	Advanced 1 CUP	Advanced 2 (Doctorate and 5 Years' Experience or More) HEJA	Advanced 2 CUP
		4.1.6 Assess the merits and limitations of qualitative and quantitative data collection for evaluation	IV.A.A2.1			4.1.7 Assess the merits and limitations of qualitative and quantitative data collection for research	IV.A.A2.1
		4.1.8 Identify existing data collection instruments	IV.A.A1.1				
		4.1.9 Critique existing data collection instruments for evaluation	IV.B.E.1			4.1.10 Critique existing data collection instruments for research	New
						4.1.11 Create a logic model to guide the evaluation process	New
		4.1.12 Develop data analysis plan for evaluation	New				
		4.1.14 Apply ethical standards in developing the evaluation/research plan	III.C.E.1			4.1.13 Develop a data analysis plan for research	New
4.2 Design instruments to collect evaluation/research data	IV.C.	4.2.1 Identify useable questions from existing instruments	New				
		4.2.2 Write new items to be used in data collection for evaluation	New			4.2.3 Write new items to be used in data collection for research	New
		4.2.4 Establish validity of data collection instruments	IV.C.E.1				
		4.2.5 Establish reliability of data collection instruments	IV.C.E.1				
4.3 Collect and analyze evaluation/research data	IV.E	4.3.1 Collect data based on the evaluation/research plan	New				
		4.3.2 Monitor data collection and management	New				
		4.3.3 Analyze data using descriptive statistics	IV.E.E.1 IV.E.E.2				

		Entry (Baccalaureate/Master's and Less Than 5 Years' Experience)		Advanced 1 (Baccalaureate/Master's and 5 Years' Experience or More)		Advanced 2 (Doctorate and 5 Years' Experience or More)	
HEJA	CUP	HEJA	CUP	HEJA	CUP	HEJA	CUP
		4.3.4 Analyze data using inferential and/or other advanced statistical methods	IV.E.E.1 IV.E.E.2				
		4.3.5 Analyze data using qualitative methods	IV.E.E.1 IV.E.E.2				
		4.3.6 Apply ethical standards in collecting and analyzing data	III.C.E.1				
4.4 Interpret results of the evaluation/research	IV.E	4.4.1 Compare results to evaluation/research questions	New				
		4.4.2 Compare results to other findings	IV.E.E.3				
		4.4.3 Propose possible explanations of findings	IV.F.A2.1				
		4.4.4 Identify possible limitations of findings	New				
		4.4.5 Develop recommendations based on results	IV.E.A1.2				
4.5 Apply findings from evaluation/research		4.5.1 Communicate findings to stakeholders	IV.E.A2.2.			4.5.2 Evaluate feasibility of implementing recommendations from evaluation	New
		4.5.3 Apply findings in policy analysis and program development	New			4.5.4 Disseminate research findings through professional conference presentations	New
Area of Responsibility V: Administer and Manage Health Education							
5.1 Manage fiscal resources	V.B.			5.1.1 Identify fiscal and other resources	New		
				5.1.2 Prepare requests/proposals to obtain fiscal resources	V.B.A2.1		

APPENDIX B

HEJA	CUP	Entry (Baccalaureate/Master's and Less Than 5 Years' Experience)		Advanced 1 (Baccalaureate/Master's and 5 Years' Experience or More)		Advanced 2 (Doctorate and 5 Years' Experience or More)	
		HEJA	CUP	HEJA	CUP	HEJA	CUP
				5.1.3 Develop budgets to support health education efforts	V.A.A1.3		
				5.1.4 Manage program budgets	V.B.A1.1		
				5.1.5 Prepare budget reports	New		
				5.1.6 Demonstrate ethical behavior in managing fiscal resources	New		
	V.D.			5.2.1 Use communication strategies to obtain program support	V.D.A1.1		
				5.2.2 Facilitate cooperation among stakeholders responsible for health education	V.D.A1.2		
				5.2.3 Prepare reports to obtain and/or maintain program support	New		
				5.2.4 Synthesize data for purposes of reporting	New		
5.2 Obtain acceptance and support for programs		5.2.5. Provide support for individuals who deliver professional development opportunities	V.D.A2.1				
		5.2.6 Explain how program goals align with organizational structure, mission, and goals	New				
5.3 Demonstrate	V.A.	5.3.1 Conduct strategic planning	V.A.E.1				

HEJA	CUP	Entry (Baccalaureate/Master's and Less Than 5 Years' Experience)		Advanced 1 (Baccalaureate/Master's and 5 Years' Experience or More)		Advanced 2 (Doctorate and 5 Years' Experience or More)	
		HEJA	CUP	HEJA	CUP	HEJA	CUP
leadership		5.3.2 Analyze an organization's culture in relationship to health education goals	V.A.E.2				
		5.3.4 Develop strategies to reinforce or change organizational culture to achieve health education goals	V.A.A1.1				
		5.3.5 Comply with existing laws and regulations	V.A.A1.2				
		5.3.6 Adhere to ethical standards of the profession	III.C.E.1				
		5.3.7 Facilitate efforts to achieve organizational mission	New				
		5.3.8 Analyze the need for a systems approach to change	New				
		5.3.9 Facilitate needed changes to organizational cultures	New	5.3.3 Promote collaboration among stakeholders	II.A.A1.1		
5.4 Manage human resources	V.C.	5.4.1 Develop volunteer opportunities	V.C.E.1.				
		5.4.2 Demonstrate leadership skills in managing human resources	V.C.A1.1				
		5.4.3 Apply human resource policies consistent with relevant laws and regulations	V.C.A1.2				
		5.4.4 Evaluate qualifications of staff and volunteers needed for programs	V.C.A1.3				
		5.4.5 Recruit volunteers and staff	New	5.4.6 Employ conflict resolution strategies	V.C.A1.5		

Competency	Entry (Baccalaureate/Master's and Less Than 5 Years' Experience)		Advanced 1 (Baccalaureate/Master's and 5 Years' Experience or More)		Advanced 2 (Doctorate and 5 Years' Experience or More)	
	HEJA	CUP	HEJA	CUP	HEJA	CUP
	5.4.7 Apply appropriate methods for team development	New				
	5.4.8 Model professional practices and ethical behavior	III.C.E.1	5.4.9 Develop strategies to enhance staff and volunteers' career development	V.C.A1.4		
			5.4.10 Implement strategies to enhance staff and volunteers' career development	V.C.A1.4		
	5.4.11 Evaluate performance of staff and volunteers	New				
			5.5.1 Identify potential partner(s)	New		
			5.5.2 Assess capacity of potential partner(s) to meet program goals	New		
5.5 Facilitate partnerships in support of health education	5.5.3 Facilitate partner relationship(s)	New				
			5.5.4 Elicit feedback from partner(s)	New		
			5.5.5 Evaluate feasibility of continuing partnership	New		
Area of Responsibility VI: Serve as a Health Education Resource Person						
6.1 Obtain and disseminate health-related information	6.1.1 Assess information needs	VI.A.E.1				
	6.1.2 Identify valid information resources	VI.A.E.1				
	6.1.3 Critique resource materials for accuracy, relevance, and timeliness	VI.A.E.3				
	6.1.4 Convey health-related information to priority populations	New				

HEJA	CUP	Entry (Baccalaureate/Master's and Less Than 5 Years' Experience) HEJA	CUP	Advanced 1 (Baccalaureate/Master's and 5 Years' Experience or More) HEJA	CUP	Advanced 2 (Doctorate and 5 Years' Experience or More) HEJA	CUP
		6.1.5 Convey health-related information to key stakeholders	New				
6.2 Provide training				6.2.1 Analyze requests for training	New		
				6.2.2 Prioritize requests for training	New		
				6.2.4 Assess needs for training	New		
				6.2.5 Identify existing resources that meet training needs	New		
		6.2.3 Identify priority populations	New	6.2.6 Use learning theory to develop or adapt training programs	New		
				6.2.7 Develop training plan	New		
				6.2.8 Implement training sessions and programs	New		
				6.2.9 Use a variety of resources and strategies	New		
				6.2.10 Evaluate impact of training programs	New		
6.3 Serve as a health education consultant	VI.D	6.3.1 Assess needs for assistance	New				
		6.3.2 Prioritize requests for assistance	VI.B.E.1				
		6.3.3 Define parameters of effective consultative relationships	VI.D.E.1				

HEJA	CUP	Entry (Baccalaureate/Master's and Less Than 5 Years' Experience) HEJA	Entry CUP	Advanced 1 (Baccalaureate/Master's and 5 Years' Experience or More) HEJA	Advanced 1 CUP	Advanced 2 (Doctorate and 5 Years' Experience or More) HEJA	Advanced 2 CUP
		6.3.4 Establish consultative relationships	New	6.3.5 Provide expert assistance	New		
		6.3.6 Facilitate collaborative efforts to achieve program goals	VI.D.E.5	6.3.7 Evaluate the effectiveness of the expert assistance provided	New		
		6.3.8 Apply ethical principles in consultative relationships	III.C.E.1				

Area of Responsibility VII: Communicate and Advocate for Health and Health Education

HEJA	CUP	Entry HEJA	Entry CUP	Advanced 1 HEJA	Advanced 1 CUP	Advanced 2 HEJA	Advanced 2 CUP
7.1 Assess and prioritize health information and advocacy needs		7.1.1 Identify current and emerging issues that may influence health and health education	New				
		7.1.2 Access accurate resources related to identified issues	New				
		7.1.3 Analyze the impact of existing and proposed policies on health	New				
		7.1.4 Analyze factors that influence decision-makers	VII.A.E.1.				
7.2 Identify and develop a variety of communication strategies, methods, and techniques	VII.B	7.2.1 Create messages using communication theories and models	New				
		7.2.2 Tailor messages to priority populations	New				
		7.2.3 Incorporate images to enhance messages	New				
		7.2.4 Select effective methods or channels for communicating to priority populations	VII.B.E.5.				
		7.2.5 Pilot test messages and delivery methods with priority populations	New				

HEJA	CUP	Entry (Baccalaureate/Master's and Less Than 5 Years' Experience) HEJA	CUP	Advanced 1 (Baccalaureate/Master's and 5 Years' Experience or More) HEJA	CUP	Advanced 2 (Doctorate and 5 Years' Experience or More) HEJA	CUP
		7.2.6 Revise messages based on pilot feedback	New				
7.3 Deliver messages using a variety of strategies, methods and techniques	VII.B	7.3.1 Use techniques that empower individuals and communities to improve their health	New				
		7.3.2 Employ technology to communicate to priority populations	VII.B.E.6.				
		7.3.3 Evaluate the delivery of communication strategies, methods, and techniques	New				
		7.4.1 Engage stakeholders in advocacy	New				
		7.4.2 Develop an advocacy plan in compliance with local, state, and/or federal policies and procedures	New				
7.4 Engage in health education advocacy	New	7.4.3 Comply with organizational policies related to participating in advocacy	New				
		7.4.4 Communicate the impact of health and health education on organizational and socio-ecological factors	New				
		7.4.5 Use data to support advocacy messages	VII.A.A1.3				
		7.4.6 Implement advocacy plans	VII.A.A1.2				
		7.4.7 Incorporate media and technology in advocacy	New				

		Entry (Baccalaureate/Master's and Less Than 5 Years' Experience)		Advanced 1 (Baccalaureate/Master's and 5 Years' Experience or More)		Advanced 2 (Doctorate and 5 Years' Experience or More)	
HEJA	CUP	HEJA	CUP	HEJA	CUP	HEJA	CUP
7.5 Influence policy to promote health	VII.D	7.4.8 Participate in advocacy initiatives	New			7.4.9 Lead advocacy efforts	New
						7.4.10 Evaluate advocacy efforts	New
		7.5.2 Identify the significance and implications of health policy for individuals, groups, and communities	New			7.5.1 Use evaluation and research findings in policy analysis	VII.D.A2.2
		7.5.3 Advocate for health-related policies, regulations, laws, or rules	New			7.5.4 Use evidence-based research to develop policies to promote health	VII.D.A1.1
		7.5.5 Employ policy and media advocacy techniques to influence decision-makers	New				
7.6 Promote the health education profession	VII.C	7.6.1 Develop a personal plan for professional growth and service	VII.C.E.1				
		7.6.2 Describe state-of-the-art health education practice	VII.C.A2.1				
		7.6.3 Explain the major responsibilities of the health education specialist in the practice of health education	VII.C.A2.3				
		7.6.4 Explain the role of health education associations in advancing the profession	VII.C.A2.3				
		7.6.5 Explain the benefits of participating in professional organizations	VII.C.A2.4				

		Entry (Baccalaureate/Master's and Less Than 5 Years' Experience)		Advanced 1 (Baccalaureate/Master's and 5 Years' Experience or More)		Advanced 2 (Doctorate and 5 Years' Experience or More)	
HEJA	CUP	**HEJA**	CUP	**HEJA**	CUP	**HEJA**	CUP
		7.6.6 Facilitate professional growth of self and others	New				
		7.6.7 Explain the history of the health education profession and its current and future implications for professional practice	New				
		7.6.8 Explain the role of credentialing in the promotion of the health education profession	New				
		7.6.9 Engage in professional development activities	New				
		7.6.10 Serve as a mentor to others	New				
		7.6.11 Develop materials that contribute to the professional literature	New				
		7.6.12 Engage in service to advance the health education profession	New				

History of Working Groups for Health Education Specialist Competency Development

Committees, task forces, and other working groups who contributed to the HEJA 2010 are listed here. Various committees of the CUP and previous committees who worked on defining the role and Competencies of the health educator are also listed.

National Health Educator Job Analysis [HEJA] 2010 (2008-2009)

Professional Examination Service
Carla M. Caro, MA; Patricia M. Muenzen, MA

HEJA 2010 Steering Committee
M. Elaine Auld, MPH, CHES; Eva I. Doyle, PhD, MSEd, CHES; Linda Lysoby, MS, CHES, CAE; Beverly Saxton Mahoney, RN, MS, PhD, CHES; Becky J. Smith, PhD, CHES, CAE

HEJA 2010 Task Force
Eva I. Doyle, PhD, MSEd, CHES (Chair); Kelly Bishop Alley, MA, CHES; Chesley Cheatham, MEd, CHES; Lillie M. Hall, MPH, CHES; Mary Marks, PhD; James F. McKenzie, MEd, MPH, PhD, CHES; Michael P. McNeil, MS, CHES; Darcy Scharff, PhD; Michael Staufacker, MA, CHES; Alyson Taub, PhD, CHES; Carol A. Younkin, RN, MA, CHES

HEJA 2010 Telephone Interview Panel
John Allegrante, PhD; Nancy Atmospera-Walch, RN, BSN, MPH, CHES; Karen Cottrell, MEd; Gary Gilmore, PhD, MPH, CHES; James Grizzell, MA, MBA, CHES; Pamela Hoalt, PhD, LPC; Jacqueline Valenzuela, MPH, CHES; Louise Villejo, MPH, CHES; Carolyn Woodhouse, EdD, MPH

HEJA 2010 Independent Review Panel
Edith Cabuslay, MPH; Elizabeth H. Chaney, PhD, CHES; Dixie L. Dennis, PhD, CHES; Marcy Harrington, MPA, CHES; Jon W. Hisgen, MS, CHES; Judith A. Johns, MS, CHES; Linda LaSalle, PhD; Garry M. Lindsay, MPH, CHES; Kimberley McBride, MPH; Larry K. Olsen, DrPH, CHES; Deyonne M. Sandoval, MS, CHES; Audrey E. Shively, MSHSE, CHES; Rob Simmons, DrPH, MPH, CHES; Cortney E. Smith, MS, CHES; Virginia Smyly, MPH, CHES; Francisco Soto Mas, MD, PhD, MPH; Jody R. Steinhardt, MPH, CHES

HEJA 2010 Pilot Test Participants
Dori Babcock, MA; Janet Baggett, MA, CHES; Christine E. Beyer, PhD; Johanna Chase, MA, CHES; Chia-Ching Chen, EdD, CHES; Lori Elmore, MPH, CHES; Brian F. Geiger, PhD; Amanda Greene, PhD, CHES; Harpreet Grewal, MPH, CHES; Brent Hartman, MPH, CHES; Marissa Howat, CHES; Bernie Jarriel, MA, CHES; Raffy R. Luquis, PhD, CHES; Grace Miranda, MA, CHES; Brandy Peterson, MPH, CHES; Tywanna Purkett, MA, CHES; Susie Robinson, PhD, CHES; Keiko Sakagami, EdD, CHES; Jennifer Scofield, MA, CHES; Jody Vogelzang, PhD, CHES; Cathy D. Whaley, MA, CHES

National Health Educator Competencies Update Project [CUP] (1998-2004)

CUP Steering Committee
Dr. Gary Gilmore, CUP Chair, Dr. Larry Olsen, Dr. Alyson Taub

CUP Advisory Committee
Ms. Elaine Auld, Dr. David R. Black, Dr. Tom Butler, Dr. Ellen M. Capwell, Dr. Helen Welle Graf, Ms. Barbara Hager, Ms. Linda Lysoby, Dr. Beverly Mahoney, Dr. Mary Marks, Dr. Marion Micke, Dr. Kathleen Miner, Dr. Sheila M. Patterson, Dr. Susan Radius, Dr. Edmund Ricci, Dr. John Sciacca, Dr. Becky Smith, Dr. Margaret Smith, Dr. Carol Soha, Ms. Lori Stegmier, Dr. Stephen H. Stewart, Ms. Emily Tyler

CUP Data Analysis Group
Dr. Randy Black, Dr. Dave Connell, Dr. Dan Coster, Dr. Gary Gilmore, Dr. Kathy Miner, Dr. Larry Olsen, Dr.Alyson Taub

Graduate-Level Preparation Standards Project (1992-1998)

Joint Committee for the Development of Graduate-Level Preparation Standards
Dr. Margaret M. Smith and Dr. Stephen H. Stewart, Co-Chairpersons; Dr. Evelyn E.Ames, Dr. Donald L. Calitri, Dr. William B. Cissell, Ms. Patricia P. Evans, Ms. Mary E. Hawkins, Mr. Douglas Rippler, Dr. Mark J. Kittleson, Dr. William C. Livingood, Jr., Capt. Patricia D. Mail, Dr. Carl J. Peter, Dr. Donald A. Read, Ms. Ruth Richards, Dr. James Robinson III, Dr. Elaine M. Vitello

Graduate Competencies Writing Ad Hoc Committee
Ms. Patricia P. Evans, Dr. William C. Livingood, Jr., Capt. Patricia D. Mail, Dr. James Robinson, Dr. Margaret M. Smith, Dr. Alyson Taub

Graduate Competencies Implementation Committee
Ms. Elaine Auld, Dr. Ellen M. Capwell, Dr. William B.Cissell, Mr. William B. Cosgrove, Ms. Patricia P. Evans, Ms. Aileen Frazee, Dr. Gary D. Gilmore, Dr. Audrey Gotsch, Dr. William C. Livingood, Jr., Dr. Sheila M. Patterson, Dr. James Robinson, Dr. Louis Rowitz, Dr. Becky J. Smith, Dr. Margaret M. Smith, Dr. Stephen H. Stewart, Dr. Alyson Taub, Dr. Elaine M. Vitello

National Task Force on the Preparation and Practice of Health Educators (1978-1988)

Chair and Founder
Dr. Helen Cleary

Vice Chair and Co-founder
Dr. Peter Cortese

Original Task Force Members
Dr. Helen Cleary, Dr. Peter Cortese, Dr. John Burt, Dr. William Carlyon, Dr. Mabel Robinson, Dr. Helen S. Ross, Dr. Warren Schaller, Dr. Joan M. Wolle

Task Force Members
Dr. William B. Cissell, Dr. John Cooper, Dr. Bryan Cooke, Dr. Robert H. Conn, Dr. Wanda H. Judd, Ms. Elizabeth Lee, Rev. Robert McEwen, Ms. Helen Savage, Dr. Becky J. Smith, Mr. Leonard Tritsch, Dr. Alyson Taub, Dr. Elaine M. Vitello, Ms. Anna Skiff, MPH, Volunteer Staff

Competency Matrices

This section contains matrices that can be used by faculty members in university programs to evaluate the degree to which their curriculum addresses the Areas of Responsibility, Competencies, and Sub-competencies of the HEJA 2010 Model. The faculty can use the completed matrices to identify specific courses in which the model components are addressed and the extent to which each Competency and Sub-competency is addressed within courses and across the curriculum. Identified gaps in coverage can be targeted for improvement. The results can be included in accreditation reports and communicated to students in the program who are interested in understanding program strengths and learning expectations.

Directions for Use of the Area of Responsibility Matrices

A matrix is provided in this section for each of the Seven Areas of Responsibility. Each Area of Responsibility matrix contains grids specific to the entry- and advanced-level Sub-competencies for that Area. It is important to remember that professional preparation for the advanced 1-level of practice should include the entry-level Sub-competencies and the advanced 1-level Sub-competencies. Professional preparation for the advanced 2-level of practice should include entry-, advanced 1-, and advanced 2-level Sub-competencies. Thus, when evaluating a program designed to prepare students for advanced-level practice, some courses will need to be listed in the entry-level grid on the matrix to indicate courses in which entry-level Sub-competencies are emphasized while other courses will need to be listed in the advanced-level grid to indicate courses in which advanced-level Sub-competencies are emphasized. It is possible that some courses may need to be listed on both grids and that some advanced-level Sub-competencies may be addressed in a baccalaureate degree.

To use the matrices effectively, enter the course number and title of each professional preparation course required of health education majors enrolled in your program. Each course should be rated only by faculty members currently responsible for its instruction. The designated course instructor(s) for a course should refer to the Competencies and Sub-competencies specific to each Area of Responsibility and determine whether or not each of the Sub-competencies is currently being taught as an integral part of the course. In making this determination, the course instructor(s) should note that a competency statement does not merely represent subject matter relevant to the behavioral skill. The statement must be viewed as an actual competency (knowledge and skills). The question each instructor must answer in connection with every Competency and Sub-competency specified in the area matrices is "Are the students taking this course merely learning associated subject matter or are they learning to perform the described Competency (knowledge and skills)?" Obviously, the instructor of each course is more qualified than any other faculty member to make that judgment.

If a Sub-competency is given major emphasis, and practice as part of a course, the instructor places the number 2 in the corresponding box. If the Sub-competency receives at least minor study and practice in the course, the number 1 is assigned. In the event that a Sub-competency is not a part of the study of that course, a zero is assigned. Figure D.1

Figure D.1. Example Area of Responsibility matrix analysis

Area of Responsibility I Matrix
Assess Needs, Assets, and Capacity for Health Education

Entry-Level

Course Title	Comp 1.1 .1	.3	.4	.6	Comp 1.2 .1	.2	.3	.4	.5	.6	Comp 1.3 .1	.2	.3	.4	.5	.6	.7	Comp 1.4 .1	.2	.3	.4	Comp 1.5 .1	.3	.4	Comp 1.6 .1	.2	.3	.4	.5	.6	Comp 1.7 .1	.3	.4	.5	Total by Course (Max = 34)*
Community Health	1	2	1	0	1	1	1	1	1	0	1	1	1	1	1	1	0	2	2	2	2	2	2	2	2	2	2	2	2	2	1	1	1	1	32
Biostatistics	2	2	2	1	0	0	0	0	0	0	2	2	2	2	0	2	2	0	0	0	0	0	0	0	0	0	0	0	0	0	0	0	0	0	10
Administra-tion of H.E.	0	0	0	0	0	0	0	0	0	2	0	0	0	0	0	0	2	0	0	0	0	0	0	0	0	0	2	2	2	2	1	1	1	1	10
School Health	1	1	1	1	0	0	0	0	0	1	1	0	0	0	0	1	2	2	2	2	2	2	2	2	2	2	2	2	2	2	2	2	2	2	25

Total by Area of Responsibility*
Should not exceed maximum (34) x number of courses

Advanced 1-Level

Course Title	Comp 1.1 Sub-comp .2	Comp 1.5 Sub-comp .5	Total by Course (Max = 6)

Total by Area of Responsibility
Should not exceed maximum (6) x number of courses

Advanced 2-Level

Course Title	Comp 1.5 Sub-comp .2	Comp 1.7 Sub-comp .2	Total by Course (Max = 6)

Total by Area of Responsibility
Should not exceed maximum (6) x number of courses

Note. 2=Major emphasis, 1=Minor emphasis, 0=No emphasis; *Maximum number possible per course

illustrates such an analysis of four health education courses. As each matrix is completed, total the recorded data to answer the following questions:

1. Of the possible number of Sub-competencies listed for the Area of Responsibility, how many are being addressed to some degree?
2. Are there any Sub-competencies or Competencies not touched upon by any course in the program?
3. Which of the courses contribute the most to achievement of the Competencies identified as essential in carrying out the Area of Responsibility?

Directions for Use of the Analysis Sheet

When all of the Area of Responsibility matrices have been completed, the analysis sheets for entry-, advanced 1-, and advanced 2-levels should be used as an organizing and summarizing tool (see end of appendix). The analysis sheets are designed to facilitate organization of the combined data obtained by means of the Area of Responsibility matrices. The same courses that appeared on the Area of Responsibility matrices are listed along the vertical axis. The data recorded on the matrices should be transferred to the analysis sheets and used to identify strengths and potential areas for improvement in the curriculum.

Notice that, for each Area of Responsibility, the Competencies are indicated by a numbering system with the first number indicating the Area of Responsibility and the second number indicating the specific Competency within that area (for example, Competency 1.1, Competency 1.2, Competency 1.3) across the horizontal axis. Below each Competency number is the total number of supportive Sub-competencies for that Competency. (See # Sub-competencies 4, 6, 7, 4, 3, and 6 for Area of Responsibility I.)

In each completed Area of Responsibility matrix, and for every course listed, enter the number of Sub-competencies given a rating of 2 and the number of those given a rating of 1 in the appropriate box (see Figure D.2). As an example, suppose that of four Sub-competencies specified as essential to the achievement of Competency 1.1 at the entry level, the instructor of a course has reported that two Sub-competencies receive major emphasis and the other two are given at least some emphasis. The number given major emphasis (in this case, 2) is entered in the top portion of the box, and the number given minor emphasis (which is also 2) is entered in the lower portion, so that it looks like a fraction (2/2). As another example, for Competency 1.2, which has six Sub-competencies, none are reported as being given major or minor emphasis. These data would be recorded as 0 (zeros) and need not be counted as they contribute nothing to the total scores.

When all of the data have been entered for all of the courses and for all Seven Areas of Responsibility, total and enter in the column at the far right of the matrix ("Course Total") the number of Sub-competencies reported as receiving major and minor emphasis with reference to each course. As you total these, include both figures of the "fraction," so that 2/2 adds 4 to the total, whereas 2/0 would add only 2 to the total. Next, total each column vertically and enter that total number in the row marked "Competency Total." The resulting "Course Total" represents the coverage of all Competencies by course. The "Competency Total" represents the coverage of each Competency across all courses in the curriculum.

Consider Competency 1.1 once again. Because there are four Sub-competencies, complete coverage of that Competency within a single course would be represented by the

Figure D.2. Example analysis sheet for the Areas of Responsibility

Analysis Sheet: Areas of Responsibility

Entry-Level

Area →	Area I							Area II					Area III			Area IV					Area V					Area VI			Area VII						Course Total^
Competency →	1.1	1.2	1.3	1.4	1.5	1.6	1.7	2.1	2.2	2.3	2.4	2.5	3.1	3.2	3.3	4.1	4.2	4.3	4.4	4.5	5.1	5.2	5.3	5.4	5.5	6.1	6.2	6.3	7.1	7.2	7.3	7.4	7.5	7.6	
# Sub-competencies →	4	6	7	4	3	6	4	6	2	4	5	4	7	5	3	8	4	6	5	2	0	2	8	8	1	5	1	6	4	6	3	8	3	12	
Course Title ↓																																			
Community Health	1*/2	0/5	0/6	4/0	3/0	6/0	0/4																												
Biostatistics	3/1	0/0	6/0	0/0	0/0	0/0	0/0																												
Administration of Health Ed.	0/0	1/1	1/0	0/0	0/0	4/0	0/4																												
School Health	0/4	0/1	1/2	4/0	3/0	6/0	4/0																												
Etc.																																			
Competency Total^^ →	11	7	16	8	6	16	12																												
Proposed New Courses																																			

Note. ***Top number:** Number of Sub-competencies given major emphasis (number of "2s" in Area of Responsibility Matrix); **Bottom number:** Number of Sub-competencies given minor emphasis (number of "1s" in Area of Responsibility Matrix)

^ **Course Total:** Sum of top and bottom numbers across all Sub-competencies for the course; **Maximum possible course score** = 162 (total number of existing Sub-competencies for Entry-Level)

^^ **Competency Total:** Sum of top and bottom numbers for all courses for designated Competency; **Maximum possible Competency score** = # of Sub-competencies x # of courses

number 4. To assess the emphasis given to that Competency as the outcome of the entire program of studies, add the reported numbers in the appropriate column. When evaluating 10 courses, the greatest possible coverage of Competency 1.1 would be indicated by a score of 40.

It is highly unlikely that any one course will encompass consideration of all of the Sub-competencies or even all of the Areas of Responsibility; however, collectively, what should emerge from the matrix survey is a graphic analysis of an existing curriculum through the 34 Competencies and the 162 Sub-competencies at the entry-level, the 34 Competencies and 42 Sub-competencies at advanced 1- level, and the 34 Competencies and 19 Sub-competencies at the advanced 2-level, as well as information regarding the depth to which each of them is being studied. The balance, or lack of it, in emphasis accorded each of the Areas of Responsibility should also be apparent.

Purpose of the Matrices and Analysis Sheets

The purpose of the matrices and analysis sheets is to provide data concerning the current degree of relevance between existing course content and that implicit in the defined Competencies; to identify strengths and weaknesses of a curriculum with regard to information; and to establish a starting point for any subsequent program revisions, adaptations, or additions. The completed analysis sheet answers most of the basic questions that curriculum decision-makers might ask about an existing program of courses in light of its potential adaptability to the competency-based plan. If more specific information is needed, the appropriate Area of Responsibility matrix will provide some answers. In other words, the horizontal matrix might show that five out of six Sub-competencies for Competency 2, Area of Responsibility I, are given only minor consideration and the other one is not covered at all. The Area of Responsibility matrix indicates which Sub-competency is omitted and which are given slight coverage. The use of the matrices and analysis sheets afford curriculum decision-makers quick answers to questions such as those contained in Figure D.3.

It is probable that the data obtained about a traditional professional preparation program in health education will show that it is not so much the content of existing courses that would have to be changed in adopting a competency-based plan. Rather, it would be a new perspective on course goals and objectives, as well as an increased use of experiential teaching-learning methods to address all Areas of the competency-based model. In any case, practice of all of the Competencies for each Area of Responsibility should be included in some instructional activity in a logically appropriate course.

Adapting existing curricula

Once the faculty has analyzed each of the courses currently offered and required of prospective health education specialists, the needed changes should be clear. Each faculty member should be charged with making the revisions necessary to better the fit between his or her course objectives and achievement of the Competencies. All faculty members should participate in planning and designing any new courses deemed necessary to facilitate implementation of Competencies currently overlooked. Though knowledge items are not used in this exercise, the validated knowledge items in Section VI of this document may be useful in course development.

Figure D.3. Sample questions for curriculum decision-making

	Curriculum Decision-Making Matrix		
Question	Findings		Needed Action
1. How many of the Competencies are currently being addressed by the curriculum?			
2. How many of the Sub-competencies receive major emphasis in the program, as shown by a rating of 2?			
3. How many of the Sub-competencies receive at least minor study, as shown by a rating of 1?			
4. If there are Competencies not now receiving any attention at all, which are they, and in what Area(s) are they found?			
5. In each of the Areas of Responsibility, how many Sub-competencies are not being addressed?			
6. Which courses are providing broadest coverage and which are providing least coverage of the Seven Areas of Responsibility?			
7. Are there any Areas of Responsibility that now receive little if any consideration in the curriculum? If so, which ones?			
8. Are there courses that appear to be irrelevant to the Competencies, as reflected in the number of zeros shown? If so, could this be changed without giving up the course itself?			
9. What implications do you see in these data for course revision, course modification, or the development of new courses?			

Developing new curricula

Where no program exists, a matrix survey would not be possible. Individuals charged with developing a brand new curriculum would start with the professional preparation curricula recommended by health education authorities, and professional groups would suggest an accepted starting point of courses to which the Competencies could logically be assigned. The validated knowledge items described in Section VI will be useful in this effort.

In arriving at decisions about where a Competency is to be taught, it is advisable to take an experimental approach. That is, decisions reached at this point need to be regarded as tentative and subject to change through trial and evaluation by students, faculty, and employers of the program's graduates. Several years of evaluation and modification may be necessary before there is assurance that the curriculum plan is providing all of the possible learning potential. Moreover, it should be remembered that the competency framework presented here is also in the process of evolution. If it were otherwise, then health education would cease to grow and develop as a discipline and as a profession.

Selecting teaching-learning strategies

It is not the function of a curriculum framework to specify or describe learning opportunities or lesson plans. Criteria for the selection of a teaching strategy include the following: (1) it must provide practice in the skill specified in the objective; (2) it must arrange for the discovery or introduction of the content; (3) the activities must be satisfying to the learner; (4) the activities must be appropriate to the past experience and present abilities of the learner; and (5) if several strategies meet the preceding criteria, the one chosen should be the strategy most likely to produce more than one positive outcome.

In general, experiential learning is more effective than passive learning in promoting competency. Everyone learns better by doing than by watching or listening. The best teaching-learning strategy is the one that encourages learners to practice doing what the objective proposes that they need to learn to do.

The Competency Framework by Areas of Responsibility

Each of the Seven Areas of Responsibility constituting the competency-based curriculum framework is introduced by a discussion of each area in Section III. A general statement is provided that describes the Area of Responsibility in broad terms: its purpose, its meaning, its application in health education practice, and its relation to the other areas.

The Competency framework for each Area is developed hierarchically as a set of Competency statements, each of which is supported by more specific and narrowly drawn Sub-competencies, upon which, in turn, measurable general objectives are based and proposed. The sequence in which the Areas of Responsibility are presented is more or less logical, but not absolute. No priorities are intended, nor should any be presumed.

APPENDIX D

Figure D.4

Area of Responsibility I Matrix
Assess Needs, Assets, and Capacity for Health Education

Entry-Level

Course Title	Comp 1.1 Sub-comp				Comp 1.2 Sub-comp					Comp 1.3 Sub-comp							Comp 1.4 Sub-comp				Comp 1.5 Sub-comp			Comp 1.6 Sub-comp						Comp 1.7 Sub-comp				Total by Course (Max = 34)*
	.1	.3	.4	.6	.1	.2	.3	.4	.5	.1	.2	.3	.4	.5	.6	.7	.1	.2	.3	.4	.1	.3	.4	.1	.2	.3	.4	.5	.6	.1	.3	.4	.5	

Total by Area of Responsibility *
Should not exceed maximum (34) x number of courses

Advanced 1-Level

Course Title	Comp 1.1 Sub-comp		Comp 1.5 Sub-comp
	.2	.5	.2

Advanced 2-Level

Comp 1.5 Sub-comp	Comp 1.7 Sub-comp		Total by Course (Max = 6)
.5	.2	.6	

Total by Area of Responsibility
Should not exceed maximum (6) x number of courses

Codes: 2=Major emphasis, 1=Minor emphasis, 0=No emphasis
*Max: Maximum number possible per course

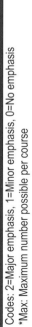

Figure D.5

Area of Responsibility II Matrix
Plan Health Education

Entry-Level

Course Title	Comp 2.1 Sub-comp					Comp 2.2 Sub-comp		Comp 2.3 Sub-comp			Comp 2.4 Sub-comp							Comp 2.5 Sub-comp				Total by Course (Max = 21)*
	.1	.2	.3	.4	.5	.6	.2	.6	.2	.4	.5	.6	.1	.2	.3	.6	.7	.1	.2	.3	.4	
Total by Area of Responsibility																						
Should not exceed maximum (21) x number of courses																						

Advanced 1-Level

Course Title	Comp 2.2 Sub-comp	Comp 2.3 Sub-comp	Comp 2.4 Sub-comp		
	.1	.4	.3	.5	
Total by Area of Responsibility					
Should not exceed maximum (8) x number of courses					

Advanced 2-Level

Course Title	Comp 2.2 Sub-comp	Comp 2.3 Sub-comp	Total by Course (Max = 8)
	.3	.1	
Total by Area of Responsibility			
Should not exceed maximum (8) x number of courses			

Codes: 2=Major emphasis, 1=Minor emphasis, 0=No emphasis
*Max: Maximum number possible per course

Figure D.6

Area of Responsibility III Matrix
Implement Health Education

Entry-Level

Course Title	Comp 3.1 Sub-comp							Comp 3.2 Sub-comp					Comp 3.3 Sub-comp			Total by Course (Max = 15)
	.1	.2	.3	.4	.5	.6	.7	.1	.2	.3	.4	.5	.1	.5	.6	

Total by Area of Responsibility
Should not exceed maximum (15) x number of courses

Advanced 1-Level^

Course Title	Comp 3.3 Sub-comp					Total by Course (Max = 5)*
	.2	.3	.4	.7	.8	

Total by Area of Responsibility
Should not exceed maximum (5) x number of courses

Codes: 2=Major emphasis, 1=Minor emphasis, 0=No emphasis
*Max: Maximum number possible per course
^No Advanced 2-level Sub-competencies exist for Area of Responsibility III

Figure D.7

Area of Responsibility IV Matrix
Conduct Evaluation and Research Related to Health Education

Entry-Level

Course Title	Comp 4.1 Sub-comp													Comp 4.2 Sub-comp					Comp 4.3 Sub-comp						Comp 4.4 Sub-comp					Comp 4.5 Sub-comp		Total by Course (Max = 25)*
	.3	.4	.5	.6	.8	.9	.12	.14						.1	.2	.4	.5		.1	.2	.3	.4	.5	.6	.1	.2	.3	.4	.5	.1	.3	

Total by Area of Responsibility
Should not exceed maximum (25) x number of courses

Advanced 2-Level^

Course Title	Comp 4.1 Sub-comp						Comp 4.2 Sub-comp	Comp 4.5 Sub-comp	Total by Course (Max = 9)*
	.1	.2	.7	.10	.11	.13	.3	.4	

Total by Area of Responsibility
Should not exceed maximum (9) x number of courses

Codes: 2=Major emphasis, 1=Minor emphasis, 0=No emphasis
*Max: Maximum number possible per course
^No Advanced 1-level Sub-competencies exist for Area of Responsibility IV

Figure D.8

Area of Responsibility V Matrix
Administer and Manage Health Education

Entry-Level

Course Title	Comp 5.2 Sub-comp						Comp 5.3 Sub-comp									Comp 5.4 Sub-comp									Comp 5.5 Sub-comp	Total by Course (Max = 19)*
	.5	.6	.1	.2	.3	.4	.5	.6	.1	.2	.7	.8	.9	.1	.2	.3	.4	.5	.6	.7	.8	.9	.11	.3	

Total by Area of Responsibility
Should not exceed maximum (19) x number of courses

Advanced 1-Level^

Course Title	Comp 5.1 Sub-comp						Comp 5.2 Sub-comp				Comp 5.3 Sub-comp	Comp 5.4 Sub-comp			Comp 5.5 Sub-comp			Total by Course (Max = 18)*
	.1	.2	.3	.4	.5	.6	.1	.2	.3	.4	.3	.6	.9	.10	.1	.2	.4	.5	

Total by Area of Responsibility
Should not exceed maximum (18) x number of courses

Codes: 2=Major emphasis, 1=Minor emphasis, 0=No emphasis
*Max: Maximum number possible per course
^No Advanced 2-level Sub-competencies exist for Area of Responsibility V

Figure D.9

Area of Responsibility VI Matrix
Serve as a Health Education Resource Person

Course Title	Comp 6.1 Sub-comp					Comp 6.2 Sub-comp	Comp 6.3 Sub-comp					Total by Course (Max = 12)*
	.1	.2	.3	.4	.5	.3	.1	.2	.3	.4	.6	.8	

Total by Area of Responsibility
Should not exceed maximum (12) x number of courses

Advanced 1-Level^

Course Title	Comp 6.2 Sub-comp									Comp 6.3 Sub-comp		Total by Course (Max = 11)*
	.1	.2	.4	.5	.6	.7	.8	.9	.10	.5	.7	

Total by Area of Responsibility
Should not exceed maximum (11) x number of courses

Codes: 2=Major emphasis, 1=Minor emphasis, 0=No emphasis
*Max: Maximum number possible per course
^No Advanced 2-level Sub-competencies exist for Area of Responsibility VI

Figure D.10

Area of Responsibility VII Matrix

Communicate and Advocate for Health and Health Education

Entry-Level

Course Title	Comp 7.1 Sub-comp				Comp 7.2 Sub-comp						Comp 7.3 Sub-comp			Comp 7.4 Sub-comp								Comp 7.5 Sub-comp				Comp 7.6 Sub-comp												Total by Course (Max = 36)*
	.1	.2	.3	.4	.1	.2	.3	.4	.5	.6	.1	.2	.3	.1	.2	.3	.4	.5	.6	.7	.8	.2	.3	.5	.1	.2	.3	.4	.5	.6	.7	.8	.9	.10	.11	.12	

Total by Area of Responsibility

Should not exceed maximum (36) x number of courses

Advanced 2-Level

Course Title	Comp 7.4 Sub-comp		Comp 7.5 Sub-comp		Total by Course (Max = 4)*
	.9	.10	.1	.4	

Total by Area of Responsibility

Should not exceed maximum (4) x number of courses

Codes: 2=Major emphasis, 1=Minor emphasis, 0=No emphasis
*Max: Maximum number possible per course
^No Advanced 1-level Sub-competencies exist for Area of Responsibility VII

Figure D.11

Analysis Sheet: Areas of Responsibility

Entry-Level

Area →	Area I							Area II					Area III			Area IV					Area V					Area VI			Area VII						Course Total^
Competency →	1.1	1.2	1.3	1.4	1.5	1.6	1.7	2.1	2.2	2.3	2.4	2.5	3.1	3.2	3.3	4.1	4.2	4.3	4.4	4.5	5.1	5.2	5.3	5.4	5.5	6.1	6.2	6.3	7.1	7.2	7.3	7.4	7.5	7.6	
# Sub-competencies →	4	6	7	4	3	6	4	6	2	4	5	4	7	5	3	8	4	6	5	2	0	2	8	8	1	5	1	6	4	6	3	8	3	12	
Course Title ↓	*																																		
Competency Total^^ →																																			
Proposed New Courses																																			

*Top number: Number of Sub-competencies given major emphasis (number of "2s" in Area of Responsibility Matrix);
Bottom number: Number of Sub-competencies given minor emphasis (number of "1s" in Area of Responsibility Matrix)

^ Course Total: Sum of top and bottom numbers across all sub-competencies for the course; Maximum possible course score = 162 (total number of existing Sub-competencies for Entry-Level)

^^ Competency Total: Sum of top and bottom numbers for all courses for designated competency; Maximum possible competency score = # of Sub-competencies x # of courses

APPENDIX D

Figure D.12

Analysis Sheet: Areas of Responsibility

Advanced 1-Level

Area→	Area I	Area II			Area III	Area IV	Area V					Area VI		Area VII	Course Total^
Competency→	1.1	2.2	2.3	2.4	3.3	*	5.1	5.2	5.3	5.4	5.5	6.2	6.3	*	
# Sub-competencies→	2	3	1	2	5	0	6	4	1	3	4	9	2	0	
Course Title ↓	**														
Competency Total^^→															
Proposed New Courses															

*Areas of Responsibility IV and VI do not contain Advanced 1-level Sub-competencies

**Top number: Number of Sub-competencies given major emphasis (number of "2s" in Area of Responsibility Matrix);

  Bottom number: Number of Sub-competencies given minor emphasis (number of "1s" in Area of Responsibility Matrix)

^ Course Total: Sum of top and bottom numbers across all sub-competencies for the course; Maximum possible course score = 43 (total number of existing Sub-competencies for Advanced 1-Level)

^^ Competency Total: Sum of top and bottom numbers for all courses for designated competency; Maximum possible competency score = # of Sub-competencies x # of courses

Figure D.13

Analysis Sheet: Areas of Responsibility
Advanced 2-Level

Area→	Area I			Area II			Area III	Area IV			Area V	Area VI	Area VII		Course Total^
Competency→	1.5	1.7		2.2	2.3		*	4.1	4.2	4.5	*	*	7.4	7.5	
# Sub-competencies→	3	1		1	1		0	6	1	2	0	0	2	2	
Course Title ↓															

| Competency Total^^→ | | | | | | | | | | | | | | | |
| Proposed New Courses | | | | | | | | | | | | | | | |

*Areas of Responsibility III, V, and VI do not contain Advanced 2-level Sub-competencies
Top number: Number of Sub-competencies given <u>major</u> emphasis *(number of "2s" in Area of Responsibility Matrix)*
  Bottom number: Number of Sub-competencies given <u>minor</u> emphasis *(number of "1s" in Area of Responsibility Matrix)*
^ **Course Total:** Sum of top and bottom numbers across all Sub-competencies for the course; **Maximum possible course score** = 19 (total number of existing Sub-competencies for Advanced 2-Level)
^^ **Competency Total:** Sum of top and bottom numbers for all courses for designated Competency; **Maximum possible Competency score** = # of Sub-competencies × # of courses

A Competency-Based Framework for Health Education Specialists – 2010

Notes

Notes

Notes

A Competency-Based Framework for Health Education Specialists – 2010